This book is dedicated to –

My wonderful husband, Jonathan and my beautiful daughter, Annabelle. I would be lost without you. Your support and love is what always gets me through.

Family and friends who supported us through my journey. No matter if it was big or small, you made a difference.

And once the storm is over, you won't remember how you made it through, how you managed to survive. You won't even be sure, whether the storm is really over. But one thing is certain. When you come out of the storm, you won't be the same person who walked in. That's what this storm is all about.

Haruki Murakami

PREFACE

Breast Cancer doesn't always strike because there is a family history. A family history has to start with someone.

In February, 2013 I found a lump in my right breast. I was 42 years old. By the end of February I had been diagnosed with breast cancer and had surgery to remove the lump (partial mastectomy) and lymph nodes. My cancer was removed.

When you are diagnosed with breast cancer you don't get time to think, or to feel sorry for yourself. You just have to make quick decisions and do what your doctors advise you. I think back now - two years later, and I can see that I was in a kind of trance, I tuned out and that was because I had no time to adjust or to allow my diagnosis to sink in. In many ways that was a good thing, especially for me at the time. The more time I had to think about what was happening, the more time I had to dwell.

Fighting the storm is my journey through breast cancer. From finding my lump, diagnosis, surgery, chemo, radiotherapy, tamoxifen and all the not so wonderful side effects.

Once diagnosed with breast cancer I was suddenly thrown into the young basket. At 42 years old I didn't feel so young and I never thought that I was too young to get breast cancer. But every doctor or nurse I saw, and even other cancer patients, thought of me as being young. It was in some ways a nice feeling but it also made me feel a little angry that in 2013 breast cancer can still be considered to only affect women over 50. That is where the awareness campaigns need to focus, in my view, raising awareness that any woman of any age can get breast cancer.

As a twelve year old only my left breast was developing, I remember my mum taking me to the doctor because she was concerned that only one breast was growing (how embarrassing) but the doctor told us not to worry, the other one would catch up! Well, it never did, all my life I have had a saggy c cup left breast and a perky b cup right breast. I'm sure that I only felt my lump because it was in my right breast, and it was easy to feel, had it been in my left breast then chances are I never would have found it.

I don't think of myself as a breast cancer survivor or a fighter. I prefer to think of myself as lucky, lucky to have found my lump early, lucky to have a team of doctors who took notice and didn't delay in the processes of finding my cancer. I just hope now that I stay lucky and it never returns.

Contents

Family History

Breast Cancer doesn't always strike because there is a family history. A family history has to start with someone.

My story wouldn't have any meaning unless I started at the beginning and mentioned my mum and sister. I am number four in a family of five daughters. There was no family history of breast cancer in my family. That was until 1995.

My sister, Annette, was 39 when we lost her to breast cancer in April, 2000. She fought so hard for 5 long years. We were all devastated when we lost her. Annette and I still lived with Mum, the day Mum and I went home without her will always stick in my memory. It was the saddest day in our lives.

Annette found her first benign lump at the age of 18. She was always the first to act if there were any changes in her breasts and always sought medical advice. In 1994, at the age of 34 she found lumps in her breast, she did the right thing by going to the doctor and specialist but unfortunately she was told that she was too young to have breast cancer, she was made to feel foolish, and the checks were not done. She was told to return in a year, that she simply had cysts.

There were so many times in Annette's life that she received the wrong treatment or doctors made a mess of it. Annette had been taking hormone replacement therapy (HRT), prior to that she had also been on the pill for years. Add high oestrogen levels and you have a death sentence. None of us knew that at the time, of course, if we had known she never would have been on it in the first place.

Finally, in 1995 doctors took notice when seeing Annette. Tests were done. I will never forget that she went alone, it's something that we have always felt sad about. I remember that she phoned Mum and told her over the phone that she had breast cancer. It was devastating news for the whole family.

Annette had surgery at Rachel Foster Hospital for Women at Redfern in Sydney. It was too late to save her breasts by then, she had a double mastectomy and all lymph nodes removed. We were told the cancer had spread to both breasts, her chest wall and her lymph nodes.

It wasn't until 2013 that I learned there were separate cancers in her left and right breasts, meaning the cancer had not only spread throughout the breast but each breast had developed its own cancer.

Annette started chemo but couldn't have more than one cycle because her body couldn't cope. She reacted badly to chemo but went on to have radiotherapy and was taking tamoxifen. But the cancer kept popping up and she never got a break. For five years she continued with treatment and had radiotherapy over and over. She had severe lymphedema in both arms and legs, the only way to relieve it was to wrap her arms and legs in cotton wool and bandages daily. Back then there were no sleeves for lymphedema, bandaging the area was the only available treatment and that did very little to help.

Annette spent a lot of time at a new palliative care hospital. Over the years she was able to go in, have a rest, stay a while and have her medications upgraded so that she was in less pain and could manage at home. We also had nurses visiting her at home to help with bathing and medications. She made a lot of friends, nurses and staff at the hospital and other patients. That hospital became her second home. She was always happy there and they took great care of her, most of the time. Everyone knew her and loved her. I would later learn in 2012 that the staff who still worked there would remember Annette and even had photos of Annette hanging in the hospital. Annette was the strongest and most caring person I will ever know. She will always be my hero. I miss her every day.

   My best friend in the whole world, my Mum, was diagnosed with lung cancer in August 2012. She was referred to the same oncologist who had years earlier treated my sister, Annette, for breast cancer. At first, she was relieved because she remembered (let's call him Dr. Neanderthal) to be "caring and nice". On my Mums first visit to see Dr. Neanderthal she was told that she had lung cancer and he would not be offering her any treatment. No chemo, no radiotherapy. My Mum was stage 4 lung cancer and was supposed to just go home and wait to die. We were told that she was too frail and having chemo may give her longer to live but it would most likely put her in hospital for most of the remainder of her life.

Mum had a mammogram and ultrasound in October 2012. One of the doctors had noticed that her left breast was indented. Mum couldn't stand for her mammogram so I was allowed to stand behind her and hold her while she had her mammogram. The technician hid behind the glass screen. For a while now I have wondered if by doing that the radiation may have caused my breast cancer. It's possible, but doesn't really matter because I would do it again if I had to. Mum was then also diagnosed with breast cancer, separate from the lung cancer.

I met with Dr. Neanderthal whilst Mum was a patient in the hospital. He had told Mum that I was welcome to speak with him and he would explain Mum's prognosis etc. When I met with him I was so upset and angry. I asked lots of questions and got answers that I didn't like. Doctors had also decided that they weren't even going to give Mum radiotherapy, nothing. To me, he couldn't care less, my opinion of his attitude was that

Mum was just another number and not a person or a mother who was loved dearly.

However, he was pushing for Mum to have a needle biopsy of the breast and a genetic test. I was told that there was a high risk that the biopsy could make Mum bleed and if she did the doctors would not act to stop it, so she would die. There was no way we were going to allow that. We couldn't see the point of more tests when they were not going to treat our mum. We were not going to risk her life for a biopsy that wouldn't give any answers to help her. Every time we tried to get some help for our mum it seemed that doors were being slammed in our face.

Dr. Neanderthal had a lot of control, even among other doctors in the field.

We lost our Mum on Friday, 7th December, 2012. In the same hospital that we lost our sister, Annette. The pain and grief I felt that day was unbearable. It was the worse experience of my life. My Mum fought hard to stay, she didn't want to leave us. I felt alone and lost the day my mum passed away. My heart remains broken.

Less than two months later I found my breast lump and was diagnosed with Breast Cancer. My doctors have told me that it was likely that I had my lump when my Mum passed. It is also possible that the stress of losing Mum caused my breast cancer.

My reaction to my diagnosis was always, why did I

have to get it now?
Why couldn't I have been given more time to grieve?

I believe things happen for a reason and I think now that
maybe getting breast cancer was the only way I was
able to get through the loss of my mum.

I was to see Dr. Neanderthal many times again after
that visit in his office. I just didn't know it at the time.

My Breast Lump

For the next two months I struggled to survive. I couldn't move past the memories of the way my mum passed away. Instead of my sisters and I coming together and supporting each other, we were barely speaking.

There were nights when I felt that I just had to get away, on my own. I remember clearly telling Jonathan that I had to leave, I couldn't stay. I just had to get away from my responsibilities and the memories. That surprised me because nothing means more to me than my little girl and husband, but I was in a very dark place and I didn't have any idea how to get out.

The weight had also dropped off me but we put it down to the stress of losing Mum.

Then, at the very start of February, less than two months after losing Mum, I woke two mornings in a row with such strong pain across my whole chest that I couldn't get up from the bed. It reminded me of when I had mastitis after my daughter was born. Each morning I had to struggle and drag myself up from the bed, then the pain would disappear. Looking back now I think it was a warning sign from above, quite possibly Mum trying to tell me to take notice of my breasts. Without the pain I'm not sure that I would have found my lump at all.

On the third morning something made me touch my right breast. As I got up from bed I gave myself a breast exam. I felt a lump. It was the size of a marble and it was painful. I played around with it for a while because I couldn't believe what I was feeling. It wasn't actually protruding, so you couldn't see it but it felt as though it was close to the surface. I could hold it between two fingers. I got my husband to touch it too, just to make sure he could feel it and he could. The first thing he said was that I had to go to the doctor. His first thought was probably the same as mine. I couldn't believe it, I had never noticed any lumps before and this was also so painful to touch.

That same day I looked at myself in the mirror and I said, "Girl, your life has just changed forever" and then I cried. I guess I already knew that I had breast cancer. At that moment there was no question in my mind. Why else would I suddenly feel a lump in my breast? What else could it be? They are some of the questions running through my head at the time. My mind was racing but I just couldn't get past what this could mean for my family, especially my little girl and that made me cry even more.

I had already, as you do, scanned the internet for information on breast lumps. Everything I looked at said that breast cancer is not painful. Great, so then I started thinking that I had a cyst, that it couldn't be breast cancer. I felt a bit silly and relieved.

On Monday February 4th 2013, I went to my doctor confident that it was a cyst or something. I explained to my doctor the pain I had across my chest and told him about my lump. My doctor did a breast exam, he found the lump almost immediately. He asked me lots of questions about my family history. Then he told me that he thought I had breast cancer. Just like that, he knew!

I look back now and my weight loss would have been a major sign. I had lost so much weight, about 10 – 15kgs.

My doctor wrote me out a referral for a breast surgeon, and sent me for a mammogram and ultrasound. He told me to ring the surgeon straight away and if I couldn't get in within 2 weeks to call and he will refer me to someone else.

My mind couldn't comprehend what was happening, instead of getting emotional, I only felt numb. I went home after seeing my doctor that day more worried about my lump but feeling as though there was still a chance that it wasn't breast cancer. I was confused and stressed about how my doctor could possibly know that my lump was breast cancer just by feeling it, before I had any tests.

I phoned to make an appointment with the surgeon. I was told to have my mammogram and ultrasound and then call back for an appointment. So, I booked my mammogram and ultrasound. I was able to get in sooner because I have a lump which was already confirmed by a doctor.

There was no point in sharing with our families at that time, so my husband and I kept it to ourselves for the time being. I was feeling desperate for my mum and was really feeling the loss. Anything I had ever been through in my life, good or bad, my mum was always there. I clung to my daughter and husband and was so glad that I had them.

I knew by going through Annette's journey with her what to expect by way of tests to confirm breast cancer. I knew that if my mammogram or ultrasound showed anything then my next step would be a needle biopsy. Until I had a biopsy it wouldn't be confirmed or definite, so I clung to that tiny chance.

Diagnosis

On the 8th February I had my mammogram and ultrasound. It was my first in about 10 years. LOL I think the smaller your breasts are the more the mammogram hurts!

Jonathan came with me and we had to wait about half an hour before my name was called. The waiting room was empty. I remember feeling very nervous and Jonathan held my hand the entire time we were waiting. I couldn't concentrate on anything, so I just sat there waiting and waiting.

Finally, my name was called, oh just my luck, it was the ladies first day on the mammogram machine. She wasn't the friendliest person I've ever met and certainly not gentle either!

I had to undress from the waist up and stand at the machine. She pulled and stretched and sandwiched my left breast in the machine. Ok, that wasn't too bad, except she was a bit rough, not only with my breast but also my body. I was told not to move for her but rather let her move me into the positions that she wanted me in. A few pictures in several different positions and my left breast was done. Now for my right breast. Not only is my right breast small but I also have a painful lump in there which just got even more painful. The lady had so much trouble getting me into position and getting my breast on the plate. To lift your arm and move your body while your breast is tightly sandwiched in a machine is near impossible and painful. Finally, after several failed attempts, we finally got it right and enough pictures were taken. I let out a long deep breath that I didn't realise I had been holding. Now, I had to take a seat, remain topless and wait while the lady went and checked the pictures she had just taken were clear enough to see.

It was at least fifteen minutes before the lady returned. She had spoken to the doctor and needed to take another picture of my right breast, "a better viewing angle". She had a film of my right breast with her which she placed up, under the light. I could clearly see my lump. I couldn't take my eyes off the film while I waited for the lady to set the machine at the angle she needed.

Right at that moment, sitting in the mammogram room, I knew for sure that I had breast cancer. I was stunned and shocked that my lump must be so large to show on the mammogram. I know mammograms don't always show up the lumps and some have been missed by the mammogram and that's why we have an ultrasound as well, for further viewing and a backup.

I desperately wanted to get out of there but I had one last battle with the lady and the machine to go.

After getting the position right and some more tugging and squishing I was finally finished. I was allowed to get dressed but still had to wait in the room until I was called for the ultrasound.

The lady doing my ultrasound was much more pleasant. As she was wiping gel over me she asked me lots of questions about my lump, how I found it and how long I've had it. As she was doing my ultrasound I could have looked at the screen but chose not to. The ultrasound was quick and painless. The lady wished me luck and I was finally able to get dressed and leave. I had chosen to pick up my report later that afternoon, rather than wait for them to be delivered to my doctor.

By this time we had shared the news with my younger sister, Georgie and my mother-in-law Beverley. Until we were more certain what the lump was we decided not to tell anyone else. We didn't want to upset or worry people for no reason, so the fewer people who knew at this time the better.

I picked up my results from the imaging centre that afternoon, I was tempted to open and read the results, which normally I would have done, but I was too scared to open it, so I waited to see my doctor.

I went to my doctor the next morning with my results. I left Jonathan and Annabelle at home and saw the doctor on my own. He went through the report with me, explaining everything. I had a confirmed carcinoma of 3cm at 11 o'clock on my right breast which had shown up on my mammogram. They suggested I have a needle biopsy. My doctor looked at the films and told me it was breast cancer. He told me the surgeon would send me for a biopsy then I would have surgery, it would all be done quickly. My doctor was very supportive and wanted to see me again after I had seen the surgeon.

When I returned home I checked my report against Mums mammogram and ultrasound reports. They were almost identical results. Both our lumps were in the right breast, mine at 11 o'clock, Mum's at 7 o'clock. Both our lumps were similar in size. Only Mum's results also showed an abnormality in her lymph nodes. Mum's mammogram didn't pick up her lump or any changes but mine did. Only Mums ultrasound had picked up her lump.

By now I was feeling exhausted. I was shocked, overwhelmed and stressed. I was trying hard to get my head around it. I really just couldn't comprehend what was happening to me. It wasn't really a matter of why me? But rather more about why now?

We updated Georgie and Beverley after my results were confirmed. It was time now to tell the rest of my family. To know how and what to say is difficult, I didn't know how to tell people, other than to blurt out "I have breast cancer". My sister, Georgie, turned 40 on Sunday 10th February. She is the baby of the family and it was her first birthday without Mum. We tried to give her a good birthday. We had beautiful flowers delivered to her and had a cake. We invited my nephew, Heath, and his family over for Georgie's birthday. Heath is our oldest nephew.

I knew I had to tell him my news, I didn't want to text or call him but I did text him that there was something I had to talk to him about. When I told him that I had "the curse", that I have breast cancer, he said he thought I was going to tell him that I was pregnant!

It was the last thing that anyone expected to hear right now. Heath said he would call his mum, my sister Tracey and tell her that afternoon.

Early that evening, Tracey text me asking if I was ok to talk. I also spoke to my sister, Sue, who offered to come down and stay if I needed her. For the next couple of days I spent a lot of time on the phone, talking and texting. It was a hard and emotional time.

All of us were in shock that this was happening especially right now, so soon after losing Mum.

It is a really hard thing to do. To tell the people in your life that you have breast cancer. It is difficult to know how or what to say. People react differently but mostly they were shocked. My sisters were all very supportive at this time, they tried to keep my thoughts positive and made me feel loved. Memories of Annette's breast cancer battle returned to all of us, it was difficult not to talk about Annette. They stayed in touch by phone calls and texts and wished me luck on my appointments.

On the 12th February 2013, I met my surgeon for the first time, Dr. Sa. He was young, about 40ish, 6 foot tall, dark and handsome. I must have had the best looking breast surgeon in Australia. He was also very charming and had a great sense of humour. He had Jonathan and I laughing a few times. He also has a stutter and anytime he says the word cancer it comes out as c-c-c-cancer.

We had an hour long visit with Dr. Sa. I remember when he asked about my family history of cancer I told him I lost my mother to cancer 64 days ago. He went silent for a long moment. He apologised to me, he said he was sorry for what I am going through. He tried to build my confidence. He was very caring during these early days. He took the time to make us feel comfortable with him and to get to know me.

He looked at my mammogram and ultrasound pictures and read the reports. He also did a breast exam. Dr. Sa confirmed that by what he could see in my reports, by feeling my lump and based on my family history that in his opinion I did have breast cancer. He could also see by the shape of the lump that it was cancer. The only certainty now was to have a biopsy to confirm my lump was cancerous and what type of cancer it was.

My surgeon told me I would have to make a decision about surgery. He gave me the option of a partial mastectomy or total mastectomy. He explained in detail the processes of each and drew diagrams of each of my options.

Option 1 - Partial Mastectomy + Mammoplasty (breast implant). My tumour and surrounding tissue would be removed and tested, along with 3 lymph nodes. The surgery is quick, I would only stay one night in hospital and I would keep my breast. Chance of recurrence is 10% over 10 years or 1% each year for 10 years. I would have a 20% chance of needing a second operation, if my lymph nodes were not clear and/or if the surrounding tissue was not free from cancer. I would have radiation afterwards.

Partial mastectomy is more extensive than a lumpectomy (is what I was told at the time). It is the removal of the area of the breast that contains cancer, some of the breast tissue around the tumour, and the lining over the chest muscles below the tumour. An implant will be inserted to replace the tissue taken and my breast will get a "lift".

A sentinel lymph node biopsy is the removal of several lymph nodes to be examined under a microscope to check for cancer cells. If cancer is found in those lymph nodes, more lymph nodes will be removed.

Option 2 - Total Mastectomy. I would have my breast removed, there would be no need for a second operation and I wouldn't need radiotherapy unless cancer was larger than 4cm. The surgery is longer and I would stay 3 nights in hospital. Chance of recurrence is 5% over 10 years.

A double/ bilateral mastectomy was not an option at the time, when I asked about it, my surgeon told me he wouldn't do it because he didn't think it was necessary.

Dr. Sa told me to think about my options over the next week and when I return for my biopsy results I could tell him my decision and plan the next step. Dr. Sa thought the quicker the whole process, the better it is for me.

I asked lots of questions about the surgery, about the need for chemo, about the chances of the cancer returning.

I wanted to know if I decided to have a partial mastectomy would he allow me to go home the same day, rather than stay overnight in hospital. I was just told that I had breast cancer but I couldn't help thinking of Annabelle. I didn't know how she would react and I wanted as little time away from her as possible.

I was about to return to the same hospital that my mother was often in and I wanted to be in and out as quickly as possible. But, Dr. Sa told me it wasn't an option, I had to stay a minimum of one night. I asked if I would need to have chemotherapy and I was told that it wouldn't be necessary unless the cancer had spread to my lymph nodes.

I was already leaning towards having a partial mastectomy and my main reason for that, I explained to

Dr. Sa, was that I have a five year old daughter who had already been through far too much.

It is so important to have a support person with you, someone who can listen and take in the information you are given. A new diagnosis of cancer is shocking and overwhelming. It is difficult to take in all the information. The minute you walk out the door it's easy to forget every word you've been told. I was very emotional and anxious. I am so grateful to have had the support of Jonathan. Jonathan was now taking extra time off work and was with me for every appointment. I just don't know what I would have done without him. I was numb and tuned out and not much information was sinking in.

Dr. Sa arranged for me to have a needle biopsy the next day and return the following week for the results and to confirm the next step.

On Wednesday 13th February I had a core biopsy at an imaging centre. A sample was taken of my lump through a needle into my breast. I laid on the bed counting the needles, some were for a local anaesthetic, I counted 7 altogether. I forced myself to look in the opposite direction until the last needle. I made the mistake of looking. The doctor asked the nurse for the 12 inch and I saw the size of it! Then I had to hold my breath, not panic and just wait for the needle to be inserted in my lump, wait for the click sound when the tissue was removed. I had a local anaesthetic but when it came to that last needle and the removable of tissue, I felt it. It was painful and I was told to prepare for the pain to worsen once the anaesthetic wore off. I had an excellent nurse and doctor who were both so gentle and caring. The doctor returned to my room before I left to wish me the best. I now had to wait until my next appointment, in a week, with Dr Sa to get the results.

By now everybody in our circle knew that I had breast cancer, most people were shocked. We had also explained to Annabelle that Mummy had a sore booby and would be going into hospital to make it better. She was scared and worried, but I did my best to comfort her. It was very important to us that she would feel confident that I was going to be alright and there was nothing for her to worry about. She was too young and still very anxious so we decided not to mention the C word. At five years old children are just too young to understand what cancer is and in my opinion they are too young to even hear that word, unless it is absolutely necessary, but in my case she didn't have to hear it, not yet anyway. She related hospital with death, if you go to hospital you die, so we had to ensure that she understood that mummy will be coming home as soon as possible. I made sure that if ever I cried that I did my best to hide it from her. Annabelle is very perceptive, if I showed any stress or fear then she would catch on straight away. Nothing was more important to me at that time than to know my little girl was alright and she understood that although I was sick, I would be coming home feeling better.

To my amazement, Annabelle went to school and told her classmates and teachers that "Mummy was going to hospital to have her booby cut off". I had no idea until one of her teachers passed me in the playground and asked me how I was doing and told me what Annabelle had said. By the end of the day it seemed the whole school knew, at least all the teachers did anyway. Teachers and parents were wishing me well. Other parents that I had become friends with since Annabelle had started school were so very supportive and offered to help us any way they could. Some of those parents have become very good friends of ours, especially Lisa who I now consider a friend for life. Lisa is one in a million, one of those people who you just know you can count on no matter what. She has a heart of gold and would do anything for anybody. She supported me and showed true friendship when my mum passed away and now she was about to do it again.

The next week was extremely stressful. I had a very hard decision to make. Should I have a partial mastectomy or full mastectomy? I had a week to decide exactly what I wanted to do. I really tried to concentrate on what method would be best for me and my family. I desperately wanted to make the right decision.
Every day, I spoke to or text family or friends, everybody was staying in touch. Almost everybody I

spoke to had an opinion. One after the other people told me what they would do if they were in my situation. The majority would just have their boobs removed or at the very least they would have one removed, as if it had nothing to do with having cancer and it was only about the breast.

I started explaining over and over again my reasons for leaning towards a partial, many times I was told by others that I was doing the wrong thing. It started driving me crazy and it was so upsetting, until finally I started standing up to people and telling them that they are not in my situation and until they are then they don't know what they would do.

Anybody, in this situation has to do what is best for them and that is what I was trying to do. I know that the people giving me their opinions and advice weren't doing it for any other reason than to be helpful or supportive but unless you have been faced with breast cancer then you really can't understand what a difficult decision it is to make. Most people assume the difficult decision is based on appearances and the fact that you don't want to lose your breast when in fact that has very little to do with it. For me, it was all about being healthy and staying healthy. I needed to do my best to ensure I would be here for a very, very long time yet.

On the 19th February 2013, I returned to Dr. Sa for my biopsy results and to plan my surgery. Dr. Sa read my biopsy results to us which confirmed cancer.

The confirmation of my diagnosis came as no surprise, after all I had basically been told from day 1 that it was cancer. But, there was no turning back now, my life had changed. I had been holding on to the minute chance that my lump could still be a cyst and the doctors were wrong, but at this moment it was absolute.

I told Dr. Sa that I had decided to have a partial mastectomy, I felt as though that was the best option for me. I knew that if he didn't get clear margins or if my lymph nodes were not clear then I would be returning for more surgery, that's the chance I had to take, I had to go with my gut feeling. I knew though that I would be having a full mastectomy if I had to return for surgery. Dr. Sa went through the process with me again. I would be having radiotherapy after I healed from surgery and I would be staying one night in hospital. We went through my reasons for deciding on a partial. They were-

I wanted to be in and out of hospital as quickly as possible. I needed to make sure that Annabelle's life was disrupted to a minimum. I was extremely anxious about that and couldn't think of anything else at that time than making sure my little girl would get through this.

Taking into account the size of my lump and the fact that my doctors were confident that I had caught it early, I was hopeful that a partial would be enough. I was too scared to think beyond having a partial. I felt that a partial mastectomy was all I could cope with. I really felt as though none of this was sinking in, I felt like a robot and making decisions like this was extremely difficult and stressful. It was happening so quickly that I couldn't get my mind around it.

I also asked Dr. Sa for his opinion, if he thought I was doing the right thing. He told me he couldn't tell me what to do but if I was his family he would suggest the partial. So then I was confident that perhaps I had made the right decision.

Dr. Sa booked me in to have a c.t scan and bone scan the next day. If those results were clear we would go ahead with surgery on the 27th February. I also had to book into hospital for my surgery. My surgery was going to cost $5500 upfront, I would be able to claim part of it back through my health fund and Medicare after my surgery.

On the 20th February, the day after my diagnosis was confirmed, I returned to the imaging centre where I had the biopsy to have my c.t scan and bone scan. Annabelle and Jonathan came with me but had to stay in the waiting room. For some reason I was only nervous about the bone scan, I thought the c.t scan was a straight forward scan that I had had before. Nothing was explained to me, I was just told "follow me", "have a seat", "put the gown on" etc.

I had to dress in a gown and have bloods taken then had a cannula inserted in my arm. I was taken into the scanning room, had to lay on the bed and I was placed on a drip of purple dye. I was told that I would feel a rush of heat, especially to my head.

The scan took approximately an hour, it included a brain, pelvis, soft tissues and chest scan. I was terribly stressed about it because I am claustrophobic and I was scared that I would be closed in the machine. It was a full body scan so I just closed my eyes when it was close to my head. It wasn't until I was finished that I realised that I had just had the c.t scan, the entire time I thought it was the bone scan.

I was sent back into the tiny change room and told to wait until I was called. I had to wait and have more dye injected into me. When I was waiting in the change room I broke down, I cried uncontrollably for the first time. It all became too much and I felt as though I just couldn't have a bone scan after just having the c.t scan. I was scared. All sorts of thoughts were going through my head. As much as I tried to control my tears I just couldn't. I couldn't stop. After about 15 minutes waiting in the dressing room the doctor finally called me. He took one look at my red face and knew I was crying. I told him that I had just received my diagnosis yesterday and having the c.t scan and bone scan today was just too much. I wasn't given a chance for my diagnosis to sink in before having to have more tests. I felt as though everything had just hit me and I realised for the first time that I had cancer.

The doctor explained that the bone scan would take about 5 hours because he had to allow the dye to travel through my body. He told me to go home and relax for a few hours and return in the afternoon if I wanted to have the bone scan. The doctor told me the bone scan was a little better than the c.t scan but if I wanted it stopped at any time I could.

I had the dye injected and returned home for a couple of hours. By the time I returned to the imaging centre that afternoon I was more relaxed but still nervous about the bone scan. As it turned out, I had nothing much to worry about. The bone scan took about half an hour. I just closed my eyes and held my breath whenever the machine came near my head.

Later that afternoon I went to book into the hospital. I received a call the next morning advising that I had to attend the hospital the next day for a pre-surgery check. This included an EEG, blood tests, checks of my weight and height and I was asked lots of questions regarding my health. I had to attend on my own and I had no idea what to expect. There were lots of people in the waiting rooms, most people had a support person with them. I met an older lady who had already had a partial mastectomy but was returning for further surgery to have a full mastectomy because her margins were not clear and cancer was found in her lymph nodes. She was handling it well although I suspect she was terrified. That lady and I crossed paths again a few months later when we were having more treatment. I was happy to find out that she was doing really well and was on the road to recovery.

On the 25th February, two days before my surgery, I saw Dr. Sa again to discuss the plans for my surgery. I was happy to have had that final visit before my surgery. Dr. Sa helped me to feel a little more relaxed about it. I was confident that I had a good doctor and I was in good hands.

Not many people in my life backed my decision to have a partial but I had the full support of my breast surgeon and that meant everything to me. I knew that if he thought I should have a full mastectomy then he would have told me so.

Surgery

I had my surgery on 27th February 2013. My surgery was scheduled for 1pm but I had to be at the hospital by 10am. I can't really say how I was feeling. I was on edge and close to breaking down. I knew though that I had no choice but to put one foot in front of the other and keep going. I've always been a nervous person but this time I had gone beyond feeling nervous or anything at all really, I felt like a robot.

My sisters Sue and Tracey had offered to come to the hospital, but they live hours away so I told them I was ok, Jonathan would let everyone know after my surgery how I was. Sue lives 7 hours away and I thought it was just too far to travel. I didn't have Mum but I had Jonathan, he was my strength and I thank God that I had him.

Before going to the hospital we stopped by Georgie's house. I know she wanted to come with me and be there with me for my surgery but she has two boys at home and there is no one to look after them if Jonathan or I can't, so it wasn't possible. She wished me luck and hugged and kissed me, we both tried our hardest not to cry. I was glad I stopped in before heading to the hospital, we both needed to know that the other was alright. We live close to each other and I would see her tomorrow.

My first stop after arriving at the hospital was at reception, I had to tell them that I was here. Then I was sent to have a scan. It was about a half hour wait before I was called for the scan. As I was waiting I received a text from Tracey that said she was coming down to the hospital and she would be there in a couple of hours. I was really grateful to have someone from my family with me.

The nurse explained to me the reason for the scan was to light up my lymph nodes with a radioactive dye, so during surgery my doctor could easily remove 3 lymph nodes including the sentinel node which is the first node the cancer would reach. I was marked up with a black texta from my breast to my underarm. The scan was used to find the correct positions. When it was time for my injection the nurse told me I would feel a painful stinging for a minute as the dye goes in. She was such a lovely nurse, at the time she was injecting the dye she had another nurse come in to hold my hands for comfort and support. That sure was the most painful needle I have had and I am so grateful to both of those nurses that day for caring about their patients.

After getting dressed I had to head down to another imaging centre to have a breast hook wire localisation, yes it is as bad as it sounds. I had a previously made appointment there for 11am. I sat and waited over an hour for the procedure, so long that Tracey and her girls had arrived and met us in the waiting room and Jonathan had to go back to reception and inform them that I would be late returning because I haven't had my procedure yet.

Finally, I was called in to have my procedure. The radiologist explained to me what would happen during the procedure. She will find the lump using the ultrasound and insert a very fine needle into the breast with local anaesthetic to numb the area where the hook wire is to be inserted. She will then insert a fine needle into the tissue to be removed during surgery. The position of the needle is checked with the ultrasound probe. Once the needle is in the correct position, a fine wire is passed down the centre of the needle and the needle is removed, leaving the wire in place. A long piece of the fine wire is left sticking out from the breast. After the procedure, this piece of wire is taped down to the skin and the hook wire remains in the breast. A final ultrasound will show the surgeon where the tip of the wire is so the tumour can easily be removed. The surgeon will remove the wire at the time of the operation. It sounded simple enough, the procedure was meant to take no longer than fifteen minutes. However, the radiologist had six attempts at getting the hook wire into position before calling for someone else to try. Apparently, the hook on the wire just wouldn't attach to the tumour. I felt every attempt but thanks to the local anaesthetic it wasn't too painful. When it was finally in place I was able to get dressed and leave, with the remainder of the wire taped to my chest.

I was feeling very drained and tired by now and hadn't even had my surgery yet. I had been at the hospital for over three hours. I had to now return to the hospital reception and was running late for the planned 1pm surgery. I was a nervous wreck but was able to somehow hold myself together throughout the whole morning. When I returned to reception I had to update my personal details that the hospital had on record. When it came to listing my next of kin I almost lost control of every emotion I had been containing all morning. My mum was always listed as my next of kin but now I had to have her name removed. I started falling apart and had to use every ounce of strength I had to contain myself. It was another reminder of what was missing in my life and another reminder that this was the first time in my life that I had to go through something without my mum. A few tears slipped down my cheek but I clung to Jonathan for support. He was now listed as my next of kin.

We went upstairs to another waiting room where we all waited together for my name to be called. We were all feeling tense and nervous. This was where I would be leaving Jonathan and Tracey and go through the double doors for my surgery. I wouldn't see them again until after I woke up and was taken to the ward after my surgery. I was so grateful to them for being there with me. It is so sad to think of anyone ever going through that alone.

The first time my name was called was for me to see the nurse and answer some questions regarding health and previous surgeries. There was a little bit of confusion amongst the nurses where I should wait. I was sent from one waiting room to another, eventually returning to the original waiting room.

The final time my name was called was for me to go into surgery. I gave a quick goodbye to everybody and went through the double doors. I was told to change into the surgery gear of gown, hat and slippers. My weight was checked and I was led to a bed, where I waited to be transferred into the operating room. Several times I was asked the same questions, name, date of birth, and what was I having done today and what side is it on.

After a short wait my turn had come and I was wheeled into the waiting area to be prepared for surgery. Again, the same questions were asked. I met the anaesthetist who gave me the injections I needed and a nurse who put in a cannula. My surgeon came into the waiting area and went over the surgery with me one final time and checked my wire in my breast. Everybody was so caring and friendly but all I wanted to do was jump off that bed and run out of there. I wanted my mum, I wanted Annabelle. I was so close to totally losing it and breaking down that I had to fight my thoughts to keep control of my tears. It wasn't because I had cancer that made me feel that way but rather just the fact that I was here and about to have surgery that scared me so much.

It was time for my surgery. I was wheeled in to the operating room, moved onto the bed, the anaesthetic was being put into my arm when before I knew it I was waking up in recovery.

In recovery my vitals were checked and I had a nurse sitting at my bedside. I don't remember feeling any pain, just very drowsy. Dr Sa came in and told me they had removed all of the tumour and he got clear margins. Good news.

Eventually, I was taken to a ward. I felt close to tears but I held onto them. Once I was settled into my room, Tracey and the girls were allowed in. Jonathan returned with Annabelle after he picked her up from school. I don't remember much of any conversations but I will always be grateful that they were there for me before and after my surgery. They had been at the hospital all day.

My breast and under my arm were padded up but I managed to take a peak. My breast was already black and swollen, it was huge, and it reminded me of a butternut pumpkin. During the night I was in pain and could barely move my upper body. The nurses gave me lots of pain medication but I still had to ring the buzzer a few times for more. I found it difficult to breathe and had sharp pain in the middle of my chest all night. I told the nurses during the night and they got me extra pain medication and told me to tell the doctors in the morning in case it was something serious. I was on a drip of fluids, pain medication and antibiotics. I hardly had any sleep, when I did drift off my snoring would wake me up.

The girl in the bed next to me was awake most of the night too, she had a bowel operation and was also in a lot of pain. I couldn't wait for the morning so I could go home and into my own comfortable bed.

Dr. Sa's team of doctors and a nurse came by in the morning. They removed my padding and checked my breast. I had bled a little during the night and had to have some of the bandages and padding changed. The doctor told me that my surgery had gone well but I would have to return to Dr. Sa in six weeks for results. I told the doctor of my pain in the chest and without checking me or asking more about it, the nurse spoke up and said "take a couple of deep breaths and you will be fine". I thought, ok, it must be normal then to get chest pain after the surgery, so I didn't mention it again. I had to wait for Dr. Sa to come in but so far I was able to get ready to go home.

I had a wonderful nurse that came in to our room after the doctors had completed their rounds. She kept returning to have a chat to both me and the girl next to me. She changed my dressings and gave me a bag full to take home, she also gave me lots of written information regarding breast cancer, and contact info. for support groups. She also showed me some arm exercises that I should do over the next few weeks. She gave me a special pillow to place under my arm, which I was so grateful for as it really helped for comfort over the next few weeks.

When Dr. Sa came in later in the morning to see me he checked my dressing. He explained that I didn't have a drain in and he thought it wasn't necessary. I was happy about that. Dr. Sa explained that I will be very sore for a while and I should see him in six weeks unless I have any problems, then I should ring his rooms to see him sooner. He said he took a large amount from my breast but he also gave my breast "a lift" when reconstructing. Dr. Sa told me that I had a very neat cut on the underside of my breast and in a year or so that scar will hardly be noticeable. Finally, Dr, Sa said I was allowed to go home. I was thrilled, I couldn't wait to get home to Jonathan and Annabelle.

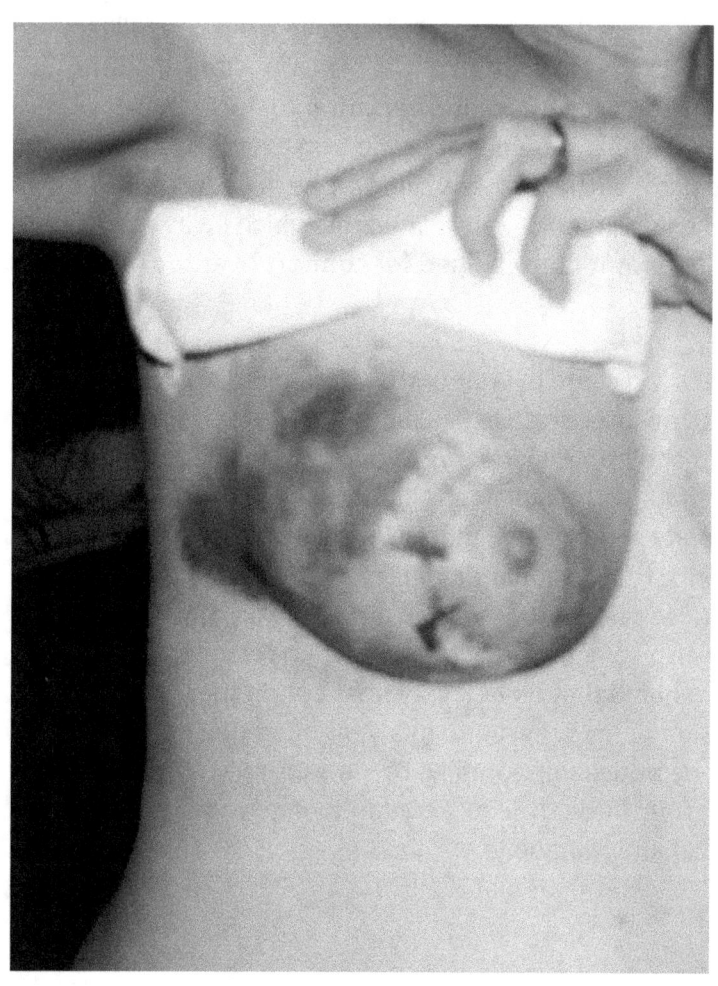

One week post surgery.

Post-Surgery

I was so excited to return home. I couldn't wait for Jonathan to pick me up. I was only in hospital overnight but there is nothing like being in your own bed in your own home. I went straight to bed as soon as I was home and I stayed in bed for most of the time over the next week. I had a special donut type pillow that I had to place under my arm, it was helping a little comfort wise but I was in a lot of pain. I was also sent home with strong pain killers, which I took and would often go to sleep after taking them. Getting and staying comfortable and pain free was the hardest. I had to use extra pillows to prop myself up. I had to be very careful when Annabelle came close or wanted to hug me that she didn't bump my breast, it was so tender and sore.

I wasn't given much information regarding care of my breast or changing of dressings. I had to just guess and do what I thought was right. On my second day home I changed what dressings I could and had my first real look at my breast. It was black from bruising and so swollen that It reminded me of a pumpkin. I had to wear a bra constantly but when I was changing dressings I knew why, the bra gave me so much support and helped ease some pain.

The pain in my chest continued over the next few days and once my pain relief medication ran out I decided it was time to see my g.p about it. I had a feeling that it just wasn't right, I was sometimes struggling to breathe and felt that I couldn't take a deep breath. The pain in my chest continued and would worsen when I took a deep breath. My doctor checked me over and started me on Ventolin and more strong pain relief but also sent me for an x-ray. He said it should have been checked when I was in hospital. I had my chest x-ray the next day and then returned to my doctor for my results. My x-ray showed that I had a collapsed lung.

My doctor told me it was caused and would have happened during surgery. I was angry that the nurse had taken no notice of me when I told her, she brushed it off as if I was just being a sook. I was also put on more medication and had to return to my doctor every two days to be checked.

I wasn't able to drive and didn't have the strength to take Annabelle to school during this time. Jonathan had taken time off work but had to return, he would still have two days where he was able to pick up Annabelle and his mum, Beverley, was able to pick her up on Tuesdays. We would have been stuck if it wasn't for other parents at Annabelle's school. They knew our circumstances and had stayed in touch after my surgery and had offered to pick up and drop Annabelle at school and then pick her up again to bring her home anytime we needed them. I will be forever grateful to them.

By week three, after my surgery, I was finally feeling close to normal. I hadn't actually been out but rather stayed home as much as I could. The swelling in my breast had gone down a lot and another x-ray showed that my lung was much better.

I felt strong enough to take Annabelle to school. I really wanted my life to get back to normal. I drove Annabelle to school and walked through the gates but I knew I wasn't able to walk down to her classroom, which was about 50 metres away, I ran out of breath and felt really tired by just walking about 10 metres. I had to have a seat and wait to catch my breath again before I could get up and walk again. I had no idea until then how much my surgery had taken it out on me, I was sure I was well now, so I was feeling a little down after that. I pushed myself a little more each day until I was able to walk all the way to the classroom.

Slowly, over the next few weeks' life returned to a new normal. My lung and breast were healing and I had gained my strength back.

Four weeks out from surgery I had another check up with my g.p, he did a breast exam and felt a large lump in the same location that my breast cancer lump had been. I knew it was there, it was quite painful but I assumed it was due to my surgery. My doctor ordered an ultrasound of my breast which showed I had a large seroma (a build-up of fluid) at the site of my previous lump. He again put me on antibiotics in case of infection and told me to show Dr. Sa my ultrasound results when I see him in two weeks. He told me I would probably have to have the seroma drained and the cause was most likely due to the fact that I didn't have any drains in after surgery. At this point I was thinking, what next?

Two weeks later I had an appointment with Dr. Sa. He did a breast exam, checked my ultrasound, felt my seroma and told me that it will be fine and eventually go away. He said draining it was not necessary. That was a relief , I was really nervous about seeing him because I knew if he was going to drain the seroma that he would do it in his rooms. He again complimented himself on my scar and the 'lift' he gave my breast. He seemed very proud of the work he had done. At this point, I took very little notice, whether I had a good scar or not was the furthest thing on my mind.

Next, we sat at his desk to hear my results from surgery and to learn the next steps in my treatment plan. After my surgery, a group of doctors came together to discuss what treatment plan would best suit me and unfortunately they had kept all of my reports from previous tests including bone scan, ultrasound, everything, so they could look over them. They were supposed to be returned to me either at the hospital or by my next visit with Dr. Sa. Somewhere, somehow they were lost and have never been returned to me. So, I no longer have any previous records or reports from any of the tests I had which could make things difficult in the future for comparisons.

Firstly, Dr. Sa told me that my surgery went extremely well with clear margins. He removed three lymph nodes and all were clear. My cancer was er+, pr+ (oestrogen and progesterone positive), meaning it was hormonal. It was stage 2b cancer.

Excellent news, at this moment I am cancer free.

Dr. Sa told me that I had a long road ahead, but he and a group of other doctors will be my side and on call to me for the next twenty or so years and will do their best to keep me cancer free.

Dr. Sa told me the likelihood of getting cancer again for me was no greater than any other woman walking around.

I was so happy and relieved, it was the best news I could have hoped for.

Dr. Sa also told me that he would now refer me to an oncologist to discuss my treatment plan, he told me she would discuss radiation, and place me on tamoxifen for at least the next five years. She would also discuss chemotherapy with me but I don't have to have chemotherapy, I can simply tell the oncologist that I won't be having it. It's an option I will be offered but it is not necessary.

Well, that wasn't exactly true. I still feel as though I was forced into having chemotherapy. Dr. Sa's opinion changed in the next few weeks and he did a complete turnaround. For that reason I no longer like going for my appointments with him, I'm not comfortable with him. My trust in him was broken.

Cancer Centre

I had to return to the same cancer centre at the hospital that Annette and Mum had been to. I was nervous about seeing Dr. Neanderthal. I knew he would be there and I didn't want to see him. Going to the cancer centre made all those memories return. I was luckier than Annette and Mum, I was referred to a lovely female doctor, Dr. Hay. However, I would have refused to see Dr. Neanderthal anyway.

On the 16th March 2013, I had my first appointment at the cancer centre at my local hospital. The same rude receptionist was still working there as when I was last there for my Mum. I sat in the same waiting area that my mum and sister had waited in. Not enough time had passed since then and I had to try hard to control my emotions as all the memories returned. I knew my doctor was a female but I had no idea what she would be like so I was nervous about that and I also dreaded seeing Dr. Neanderthal. I hoped he wouldn't be there today, I was still angry with him for so many wrongs from the time my mum was diagnosed.

As I waited for my name to be called who would walk out of his room but Dr. Neanderthal, I couldn't believe it. He recognised me immediately and hesitated as he walked past me, I think he considered speaking to me, but most likely saw the look on my face and thought better of it. He went to the reception desk possibly wondering if I was there to see him for some reason and not expecting me now to be a patient of the cancer centre that he heads. I'm sure that he was looking for my file but at that time he wouldn't have known that my surname is different because I am married.

I know these doctors see many people and patients but it had been such a short time since I last spoke with Dr. Neanderthal that I knew he recognised me. Regardless of the time gone by when mum first saw him he commented that he remembered my sister Annette years earlier.

My appointment with Dr. Hay confirmed that Dr. Neanderthal would most likely obtain information about me and could possibly look through my file, which annoyed me to say the least. I really didn't want that doctor to know anything about me and it really upset me to see him at all. It made me feel sick in the stomach that he would have anything at all to do with my treatment.

Finally, after a short wait, Dr. Hay called my name. My guess is that she is in her thirties. She is not at all your typically stuffy looking doctor. She looks just as any average person does and greeted us with a lovely big smile. She is softly spoken. Again, Jonathan was with me to meet Dr. Hay.

Dr. Hay was already familiar with my breast cancer history. She asked lots of questions about my family history and asked for permission to obtain my mothers and sisters files, since they had both been patients at the hospital and cancer centre, for further information regarding their types of cancers etc. She checked my breasts and also commented on my scar. Dr. Hay explained to us what my type of cancer was, er+ pr+, and what that meant in regards to treatment.

Having high levels of oestrogen most of my life has caused my cancer, as my cancer is oestrogen positive. I would be placed on tamoxifen for at least five years. I would go into early menopause and the treatment would block my oestrogen levels so that hopefully with lots of checks the cancer won't return. I would also have radiotherapy treatment but would see the radiation oncologist for that. Dr. Hay explained to us and showed us diagrams of other treatments available to me and the benefits they would have over the next ten years.

Dr. Hay suggested that I have chemotherapy, due mostly to my family history and to ensure there was no more cancer in my body. I was given a choice because chemo was not a necessity for me rather it was an option I was being given to take the best approach possible in ensuring the cancer does not return. Dr. Hay explained to us that with chemo, my chances of the cancer never returning would increase by a further 1% added with the other treatment that I would be having.

Nothing scared me more than chemo, I was terrified of it. I felt as though I just couldn't have it. I don't think anybody has been able to understand my fear of it. I don't know why I feel so strongly about it, only that I saw Annette have one cycle of chemo and the horrible reactions she had to it. Most people are aware of the side effects of chemo- hair loss, nausea etc. They're not the only reasons for not wanting to have chemo. My fear comes from deep within, I don't really understand it myself. I remember as a kid, thinking if I ever got sick I would never have chemo.

Dr Hay was great, I was able to explain to her my fears and we had a good discussion about it, she wasn't pushy at all and she was as honest as she could be with me. She understood about my sister and told me chemo had changed since then, it was much better now and there are lots of medications for nausea to take that really help. I told her that I didn't expect to have chemo because Dr. Sa had explained to me that as long as I was clear then I wouldn't need to have it. I said that had I known before my surgery then my decision would have been a different one. She explained to me that due to my family history and the fact that I was stage 2 it would be the best option for me.

I looked at my husband, Jonathan, and he was nodding his head yes, telling me to have chemo. Seeing the desperate look in his eyes really hurt. My thought then was, how can I not have chemo when I have my husband pleading and wanting me to do it. It didn't matter how fearful I was, Jonathan was too. I knew I had to do what was best, anything to give me a chance at a long healthy life and to be here with Jonathan and Annabelle. I had no choice but to do whatever would give me the best chance, for myself and my family. As scared as I was, I told Dr. Hay that yes I would do it, I would have chemo.

Dr. Hay told me that chemo had changed over the years, since my sister would have had it, they can better look after patients now and the reactions and side effects are much better than before. Dr. Hay made me an appointment for the following week to meet with the chemo nurse but also told me to go home and think about it some more and see her before my scheduled appointment with the nurse if I had any questions or if I decide not to go through with having chemo. She wanted to make sure I made the right decision, for me. She understood how I felt about it. I am so grateful to her for understanding and giving me the opportunity to think about it. Dr Hay didn't want me to make a hasty decision and she could see how distressed I was at the news.

I went home and thought of nothing much else for the next week. Dr. Hay was still allowing me to think about whether I was having chemo or not, nothing was set in stone yet. Once I explained to Jonathan my fear of chemo and my worries he understood and became the person to listen to me without forcing his own opinion on me. Again, he totally supported me and any decision I made, I would always have his backing. I desperately wanted to do the best for me and my family and do whatever I needed to, to be here in the future, to make sure this horrible disease never returned, but that 1% just kept sticking in my head. For me, 1% was a tiny amount, for all that I would go through with having chemo, would that 1% make any difference whatsoever? Would it be worth it?

For the next week I hit a new low. I was getting quite depressed and cried often. I was shocked that chemo was being offered when I had already been told several times before that I wouldn't need to have it. I already knew that if I wasn't given the all clear after my surgery that I would have chemo, no questions asked, but because I am being given the option of having it, because it is being offered as a precautionary measure and I have to decide to have it or not has made it such a stressful, difficult decision. I know there are people living with this disease who desperately wish they were in my situation. I went through this with my mum, we were desperate for any doctor to treat her cancer. I can't explain my fear of chemotherapy, but it has always been there. This decision was not an easy one, as scared as I am feeling I still have to do the right thing, the best thing. Suddenly, my prognosis and treatment options had changed, taken a new turn, now I had to decide what to do about it.

Once again how Annabelle would react became my main focus. If I was to have chemo we would have to tell her upfront what to expect. We couldn't hide anything from her this time. It scared me more knowing that I could get very sick, lose my hair and my daughter would see it and go through that with me. I just couldn't do it and the thought of it was making me sick. I thought about this long and hard, I didn't make my decision lightly at all, but after a week I made my decision.

I would not be having chemotherapy.

I returned to the cancer centre and Dr. Hay a week after my first appointment. For the second time Dr. Neanderthal walked out when I was in the waiting room, this time he lingered and gave me half a smile when he walked past me. At that moment I knew that he had read my file and he knew why I was here, I was even more annoyed by that. How I hate seeing that man every time I am here. I blame him for the mistreatment of both my mother and sister Annette and seeing him every time I am there is just so difficult. Seeing him brings back all the bad memories that I try hard not to think about.

I was feeling very nervous about seeing Dr. Hay. I had to tell her that I wouldn't be having chemotherapy and I wasn't sure how she would react. When Dr. Hay called me into her room I think she already had an idea that I would be telling her no to chemo. She could see that I was quite stressed and asked me if I was o.k. I told her my decision and my reasons for coming to that decision. Dr. Hay told me that's fine. She told me I shouldn't have worried so much and the reason it was so difficult was probably because it was an option, a precautionary measure. I was so relieved, she made me feel as though it was O.K. to say no. She made me feel as though even without chemo I would still be alright. Dr. Hay told me I would still have radiotherapy and take tamoxifen for the next five years, possibly ten years.

Dr. Hay wrote me a referral for an appointment to see the radiotherapy oncologist so that I could get started on radiation as soon as possible. She also wrote me a script for tamoxifen but told me to start that after radiotherapy has finished. I would return to see Dr. Hay in three months.

Until I had spoken to Dr. Hay I still wasn't sure if my decision would be the right one. The decision to have chemo or not was basically left to me. As strong as my fear is of chemo had I been told from the start that it was necessary as part of my treatment plan then I would have somehow prepared myself and would have had chemo, definitely, because it would help to save my life. I was placed in a difficult situation to decide myself. Not all cancer patients get the chance to have an option as part of their treatment. Like my mum not all patients are offered treatment. People can say that I was lucky to have an option but to me being in that situation just made things harder and more stressful.

I was happy now that my decision was the right one for me and my family. All the stress of the past week had been lifted. My next step was to start radiation therapy.

When your plans are changed

I had my first appointment with my radiotherapy oncologist Dr. Brown in March, 2013 at the cancer centre. Dr. Brown wasn't able to attend because her daughter was sick so I saw one of her registrars. She did a breast exam, asked me questions regarding my surgery and treatment so far. We discussed my decision not to have chemo and again, she was also understanding. I felt as though I had the support of my doctors so I was feeling confident that my decision not to have chemo was the right one for me.

She asked questions about radiotherapy, was I prepared to have it? It's a lot easier than chemo but I will be left with burns like a suntan. I was comfortable about having radiation, I had taken Annette to her radiation appointments and although I hadn't seen the actual machines I knew that it was a painless and quick process. I was given the paperwork and told that I would have radiation at a different hospital because my local hospital doesn't provide it. I would have it every day for nine weeks, a total of 43 times. Once the doctor knew I was ready for it I was booked in to the hospital for an appointment. The doctor said the hospital will call me later that day with my times and dates. The first step in having radiotherapy is to have the area tattooed and scanned. I left that appointment feeling less stressed and ready to start my next step.

Unfortunately, that feeling wasn't going to last long.

By that afternoon, within a few hours of leaving the doctor and the cancer centre, I had fifteen phone calls from doctors, receptionists and councillors. My mobile and home phone were sometimes ringing at the same times. As one person was speaking to me another was continually calling, trying to get in touch with me on the other phone. I couldn't believe what was happening, just when I started relaxing and feeling like I can do this everything was just about to change.

My first call was from the cancer centre at the hospital. An appointment was made for me to go the following week and have scans done to mark up where I would be having radiation, as discussed in the morning with my radiation oncologist. Too easy, I was feeling good about getting started, the sooner I started the sooner I finished and I could start getting my life back to a new normal. Once I get marked up then I will begin my radiation therapy.

The moment I hung up the phone it rang again. It was the doctor that I had seen this morning. Apparently, the doctors had a meeting this morning to discuss my treatment plan. I'm still not sure who "the doctors" might be but I can guess that one of those was most likely Dr. Neanderthal as he is in a position of authority within the cancer centre. I was told that "the doctors" had gone through my file and discussed the best options for me. During this meeting, that I was never aware of, "the doctors" decided that I wouldn't be having radiotherapy, it was being cancelled. Instead I will be booked in for a genetic test. I was told that I would have the genetic test first, if it came back that I was positive to the gene mutations of BRCA1 or BRCA2 then I would have surgery to remove my breasts. Therefore, radiotherapy would not be necessary. If I was negative to the gene mutations then radiotherapy would be rebooked.

To say I was angry is an understatement, I was outraged. I couldn't believe what I was being told. I wasn't being asked what approach I would like to take nor was I asked if I wanted to take a genetic test. I was being told. The doctor was only a registrar so was basically just passing on the information to me from "the doctors" so there was no point in telling her MY views, I wasn't getting anywhere. She basically wanted to tell me that the genetic councillor will be calling me this afternoon to discuss the genetic test with me. I told her that my appointment had already been made for radiation and she told me that it will be cancelled.

This smelt of Dr. Neanderthal. He was so pushy in trying to get mum to have the genetic test and now it was my turn. I don't understand why. Why is it so important to the doctors at the cancer centre for patients to have the test regardless of their prognosis being good or not. My own Dr. Hay never mentioned the genetics test and she works at the same cancer centre. This was the confirmation to me that although I wasn't a patient of Dr. Neanderthal he had access to my records and could even make decisions on my treatment. I was not comfortable with that at all.

A few moments after hanging up from the doctor the councillor phoned me. I really didn't get the chance to let this sink in. I told the councillor that I felt like I was being forced into having the genetic test. She wasn't aware that my radiation appointment has been cancelled. I explained how angry I was about the decisions being made for me. The councillor told me I could take some time between now and when the appointment is made for me to think about whether I will have the test or not. The councillor told me that this is totally my choice and if I don't want to have it then that's fine.

She asked me lots of questions regarding my family history of breast cancer and other cancers. I was expected to know my full family history including relatives I have never met or never knew. There were many questions I couldn't answer simply because I didn't have the answers. It was very personal. It felt like they were digging too deep. The councillor agreed to call me again in the next couple of days, to give me the chance to find some answers to her questions. For that, I had to contact my cousin, Cheryl, the only relative on my mum's side who I have heard from since Mums death. Out of all of my distant relatives, she is the only one I have a relationship with and the only person I would want to discuss my situation with.

The phone calls kept coming, that afternoon. Doctors and receptionists changing my appointments and trying to explain to me their reasons for the decision they made that day. Dr. Brown, the radiation oncologist, also called me to explain the situation. I didn't feel like I had any choice but to accept their decision but that didn't stop me letting them all know how I felt about it and how wrong I thought it was. I was adamant that regardless of the results of my genetic test, the decision to have any future breast surgery is mine and mine alone and I will not be forced into that.

As helpful and as knowledgeable as medical staff are it is important sometimes to take a stand. Some decisions cannot and should not be made for you. Throughout my diagnosis, surgery and treatment, I asked lots of questions and made sure I had a good understanding of my situation through the eyes of my medical staff. Everybody wants to do what is best for themselves and have the absolute best outcome. By questioning your medical staff and obtaining as much information from them as possible about your diagnosis and their plans for your future won't harm anybody. If you have medical staff who don't explain things to you or don't answer your questions, then it is ok to get a second opinion if you're not comfortable. This is your life and you want to get the best from your medical staff as possible.

I called my cousin Cheryl and explained to her that I have breast cancer. We chatted for a little while about that. She was shocked to learn my news. I asked her not to tell any of our relatives. I would do it later when the time was right for me, most likely only if I tested positive to the gene mutations. I was still angry and upset with some of my mother's sisters and her brother, only two of them bothered to go to mums funeral, none of them visited her at home or in hospital when she was diagnosed. My mother was one of 12 children, at the time of my mother's death 7 were still living, they all also had children, so we come from a very large family. Cheryl was the only person to visit with mum in hospital. None of us, to this day have had any contact with my mums family since her death, except Cheryl and my Aunt Shirley. My mother deserved better from her relatives, until her illness she was in regular contact with them, none of the relationships were strained. People stayed away, knowing her condition, they cut all ties with us the moment they heard Mum was sick and that continues today. If I was to test positive to the breast cancer gene mutations I would feel obligated to tell my mums relatives. If I don't have the gene mutations then there is no reason for any of them to know.

I knew Cheryl was the go to person regarding information about our grandparents' medical history. I needed to find out exactly what they died from. I already had the information about our Grandmother because Mum often spoke about her. She died at the age of 60 from a stroke or cerebral haemorrhage. But I wasn't sure about our Grandfather and I knew that Cheryl would have that information. I never knew my Grandparents but Cheryl had grown up having had relationships with both of them. It turned out that our Grandfather and two of his relatives had all passed away after having stomach cancer. This was important information that I had to pass onto the genetics councillor.

The genetics councillor called me again after a few days. I gave her the information that I had obtained. I also lost an aunt to leukaemia just a few years ago. It seemed any cancer in the family was all on my mother's side. As far as I know there is no cancer on my father's side. It was a difficult conversation to have. It raised many sad memories for me, having to recall dates of diagnosis and deaths for my loved ones and the reasons for their deaths. Speaking of my dad was extremely difficult, I felt that it was irrelevant to my situation but the questions still had to be answered. I told the councillor that I lost my dad on the 23rd September, 2000. Two days before what would have been Annette's 40th birthday and just six months after Annette passed away. My dad was coming home from shopping, walking on the footpath to the bus stop when an out of control car mounted the footpath and ran him down. My father died at the scene. We never got the chance to say goodbye. I still struggle talking about it, it was such a difficult time in my life. Losing him ripped my heart out.

  The councillor made an appointment for me at the genetics centre at Royal Prince Alfred Hospital in Sydney. I was told that due to my family history of breast cancer, me being the third woman diagnosed with breast cancer in my immediate family, then we are considered high risk for the gene mutations BRCA1 and BRCA2.

I took the appointment but I planned to think about what steps I would take. I was so upset, this felt like yet another road block. Right when I thought I was able to get through this and the hardest parts were behind me, this happens. I had already planned with my surgeon, Dr. Sa to have the genetic test once I had finished with my treatment. In his opinion, at the time, it was more important to complete my treatment first, once that was over, then he would send me for the genetic test.

That made sense to me. Now, with these latest developments, I took several steps backwards emotionally. I was feeling depressed, confused and emotionally drained. Before committing to the genetic test I planned on speaking with Dr. Sa at my next appointment which was in the following week.

When Trust is Broken

It was now the start of April, 2013. My breast was healing and was starting to look more normal, with the bruising subsiding and the swelling going down. My appointment for the genetic test and counselling was set for the 4th of April.

I was more down and depressed than I had been throughout this experience. The events of the past weeks had really upset me. I couldn't wait to see Dr. Sa and discuss with him what has been happening.

On the day of my appointment I sat in Dr. Sa's waiting room. I must have looked as bad as I felt because his receptionist asked me if I was o.k. I expected Dr. Sa to back me up, based on our previous conversations, I was about to find out how wrong I was.

Dr. Sa called me into his room. I sat down and we started the conversation. Firstly, I spoke with him about the incidents of the past week or so. How my radiation was cancelled and I felt like I was being forced to have the genetics test. Suddenly now there was no rush for radiation and he said I should go ahead and have the genetic test. He spoke like it was no big deal.

Apparently, radiation can be done at any time. He did explain to me that once I have radiation therapy on my breast, it will be more difficult to have reconstruction on that breast due to the damage radiation causes. He said I am probably better off having the genetics test first and then making the decision once I have the results back. He did stipulate that it was my choice and only I could make that decision of whether I would have a double mastectomy or not. So, I did get a little bit of support from him.

Now, Dr. Sa mentioned chemo. I wasn't expecting that topic to come up because the decision had already been made. I told Dr. Sa that I wasn't having chemo and I had already discussed it with Dr. Hay but Dr. Sa, unknown to me, was already well aware of it. Remembering that this same doctor is the one that told me I wouldn't be having chemo in the first place. I spent two hours in his room. He asked me my reasons for not having chemo and I explained to him exactly why I couldn't have it. Dr. Sa asked me if I was scared of chemo and I said yes, yes I am scared of chemo. I then went through my other reasons for not having it.

1. I'm told that it is an option for me that combined with other treatment will increase my chances of the cancer not coming back by 1%. To me 1% is not reason enough to have chemo.
2. When considering chemo I also had to think about how it would affect my daughter. I strongly believe that she has seen too much and

has been through too much for a five year old. I am scared of the effects it will have on her.
3. I was told from the start that I wouldn't need chemo.
4. I thought long and hard and I believe that I have made the right decision for me.

After hearing my reasons for not having chemo, Dr. Sa told me that it was just "a cop out". I was so shocked at his attitude. I didn't know what to say.

Jonathan and I sat in his room for two hours, it was the longest lecture I have ever received in my life. Dr. Sa. was angry and he made sure I knew it. I was "stupid" for not having chemo and my reasons were just "excuses". When I started crying and tried defending myself he continued on his rant. He told me that the 1% should be looked at in other ways. What got to me the most was when he said that some people would do anything for the chance to be offered chemo. To be given any chance of survival. For some people being offered a chance of 1 percent is enormous and I should think about how lucky I am to be offered this chance. He told me that chemo was nothing like I seem to think it is. There are so many medications now to help with the side effects and the doctors will watch me closely daily.

I will never forget that day and the way Dr. Sa spoke to me. Since that visit I have felt nervous on every other appointment with him. My trust was broken that day. Here is a doctor that I felt so comfortable with and relied on to give me the best advice. To tell me my reasons for not having chemo were just a cop out really upset me. I tried to remind him that he told me from my very first appointment with him and every visit since then that I wouldn't need chemo but he didn't want to hear anything I had to say. I reminded him that I know too well what it feels like to be told there is nothing to be done. I also tried to remind him how many times he has told me that my cancer was caught early. Now, he was making me feel like I would die without chemo. It was a total backflip on his part and I really even now don't think most of what he said to me that day was necessary. Looking back now, I think I should have walked out on him that day and sort a new surgeon. Obviously, I wasn't my normal self or in a good place and as my doctor he should have seen that. Nobody should ever be treated the way I was that day.

Dr. Sa wanted me to change my mind that day in his surgery and that is exactly what I did. I was left feeling as though I had no choice but to agree to have chemotherapy. I had never taken my decisions lightly but now I was feeling so scared that the information I was given previously was incorrect and my only choice now was to have chemo. I always said that I would do what was best for my family and do what would give me the best chance.

Genetics Test

On the 4th April, 2013 Jonathan and I attended the Cancer Genetics Clinic at The Royal Prince Alfred (R.P.A) Hospital in Sydney. The clinic is located inside Gloucester House. The same building where Annette had received some of her treatment, before moving to the hospital closer to home. Back then, I saw it as a very old, creepy, dilapidated building, set back far off the street. It was a horrible place, and I disliked going in there. It looked like a building that had a very poor, scary history and the last place cancer patients should be.

The moment we stepped inside the building it became familiar to me, little had changed. We got in the old rickety lift and went to level 2. We had a short wait, waiting to see the councillor and doctor. I felt sad being in that building again and I sat remembering the times I had been there years earlier with Annette and Mum.

I was to learn that there were two doctors with the name Annabelle and a councillor with the name Georgina. I wasn't to meet all of them but we had a laugh about such unusual names that belong to members of my family also belonging to staff at the genetics clinic.

First, we met with the councillor, the same girl that I had spoken to on the phone. I again exchanged information with her regarding my family history of cancers.

On my mother's side –

My Great Grandfather – Carcinoma Stomach
Grandfather – Carcinoma Stomach
Grandmother – Cerebral Haemorrhage
Great Grandfather – Cerebral Haemorrhage
Aunty – Leukaemia
Aunty – Crohns Disease
Uncle – Prostate Cancer

There is no known cancers on my father's side.

Then there is –

My Mum – Lung Cancer and Breast Cancer Aged 77
Sister – Bilateral Breast Cancer Age 35 at diagnosis
Self - Grade 2 infiltrating ductal carcinoma er+ , pr+ , her-   Age 42

We then discussed, with diagrams, how cancer forms, our genetic makeup, faulty genes and testing.

I had to sign and agree to the clinic obtaining Annette and Mums records. As Annette had been a patient there, her records would still be there.
  We met with the doctor who explained the test to me. My family history was assessed to determine the

likelihood of an inherited mutation in one of the breast cancer genes, known as BRCA1 and BRCA2. The likelihood of detecting a mutation was over 10%. I was the most appropriate person in my family to have the test as I have been diagnosed with breast cancer. Therefore, I agreed to have the test, a blood test, to be taken whilst I was there. She was going to rush it through to allow me to start my radiation ASAP. As my family were determined to be at a potentially high- risk, if I test positive to the gene mutation then my family will also be tested at a later date. We expected to receive the results within 2 – 3 weeks' time.

Chemo

Now that I had agreed to have chemotherapy, I had to
make another appointment to see Dr. Hay. I saw her
again on the 9th April. I was a little embarrassed because
I had changed my mind about having chemo so many
times already. I explained to her why I had changed my
mind this time and my visit with Dr Sa. She was so
pleasant and very understanding. All doctors should
have her manner, it makes life with cancer that much
easier to have a good doctor. I explained to her that all
along, all I've wanted to do is what is best for my family.
I told her my fear of chemo was real. Dr. Hay suggested
that I at least have the one cycle and if I want to I can
stop after that. I felt comfortable with that, I was
prepared to at least have the first cycle and go from
there.

   Dr. Hay booked me in to see the chemo nurse, Shaz,
she would explain all the details to me and take care of
me. She wrote out scripts for all the medications I would
be needing, including extra nausea medication because I
suffer from motion sickness. I had to also have a blood
test before chemo started. Dr. Hay understood how
nervous I was so she also gave me a script for a
medication to help my nerves on the day of chemo. I
needed to take one tablet an hour before chemo. Again,
I was reassured that I will be looked after, closely
monitored and most importantly, chemo was much
better now than in the past, it isn't as nasty as it once

was. I was to learn that statement was so incorrect, in my case anyway.

Had I known at the time what chemo would do to me I never would have agreed to have it, whether I was virtually forced into it or not. No-one would have changed my mind. I was scared and had a real fear but I had no idea what chemo would do to my body.

I met with Shaz the chemo nurse two days later. She was very friendly and caring. Shaz explained chemo to us. I would be having Tc chemo a mix of Docetaxel and Cyclophosphamide. I would have it every three weeks and I would have four rounds or cycles. I would have to have a blood test the day before every new cycle to check my blood count is normal. Shaz explained how to take the medication and when to take it. I was given paper work to take home and read regarding side effects and what to expect on chemo. I was told my hair would start to fall out after the first dose, within one to two weeks. Although, the list of side effects were given to me, they were immediate side effects, no-one mentioned what the long term side effects could be. I also wasn't told that my doses of chemo are very strong, I would, however, be told afterwards.

Shaz took us to the chemo rooms and booked me in for Friday 19th April at 11.00am for my first cycle of chemo. It would take about five hours, at least for the first dose as it has to be administered slowly. I was given gloves that I would have to put on before putting my hands in ice to prevent my nails from turning black. I was given a card so I could get free parking for the next three months.

I remember snippets of this time but mostly I think I was too robotic and spaced out to take in all the details. In my mind, I was about to experience the scariest moment of my life. How I would get through it I had no idea, only to say sometimes you do things and get through them only because you have to. When you have no choice, then you go with the flow, even if in a state of shock or trance like. My job now was to convince myself that this is the best thing for me to do. I had only a week to prepare myself and my daughter for what was ahead of us.

The first thing I had to do was tell my little girl, who was still only five years old, that I would be having chemo and prepare her for that. We had to tread carefully only giving her enough information so that she would understand what was going to happen. However, at this time we had no idea ourselves what would happen. We told Annabelle that mummy had to have some medicine that is going to make my booby better but I might get a little bit sick first.

When we told her that I would lose my hair we turned it into something fun, so she wouldn't worry too much. I had long, very thick, curly hair. I didn't want my hair falling out in big long clumps. I knew if Annabelle saw that, that it would scare her and I was worried about how to approach it. I knew that I would lose my hair soon after having chemo, so I made an appointment at the hairdresser and took Annabelle with me to get my hair cut off. We went for a number two haircut all over, just leaving a long fringe, which we then let Annabelle choose a colour that she wanted put in. Annabelle chose pink and purple. For the first time in my life I had short hair and a pink and purple fringe. It was a fun moment for both of us. I had no idea, because I always thought I had a big head, but the hairstyle suited me and as it turned out my head shape was perfectly round. Getting my hair cut before having chemo was one of the best things I could have done.

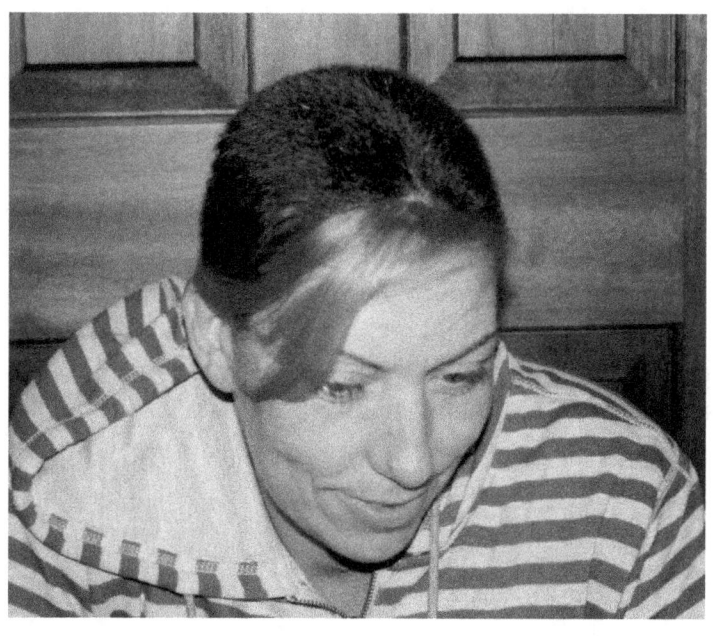

Some people are comfortable wearing a wig when they lose their hair, others are comfortable showing off their baldness. I knew that I wouldn't be comfortable with either of those choices. I decided to wear beanies and hats, just like my sister had done when she lost her hair. Both Annabelle and I went shopping for beanies and hats. To make sure my head would be covered I went for the slouch beanies in a feminine style. Of course, pink being Annabelle's favourite colour we bought pink beanies. I also purchased cotton open ended pieces to wear under the beanies for comfort mostly so that the beanie wouldn't annoy my bald head. We also got a couple of long scarves just in case the beanies were no good. These were to be my birthday present that year as my 43rd birthday was on the 14th April, five days before I would start chemo.

I developed a chesty cough and a cold a few days before I was due to start chemo. I had an x-ray and was put on antibiotics. My local doctor expected that chemo would be cancelled. I had to tell the chemo nurses on the day of chemo.

The day before my chemo I had to have a blood test at the hospital to make sure my bloods were ok to go ahead with chemo. I also had to begin taking medication, dexamethasone, to help reduce the side effects of docetaxel. Dexamethasone helps to reduce the amount of fluid retained in your body and would also help with nausea. I noticed a change almost immediately. I was hungry, felt energised and couldn't sleep.

The day of chemo arrived so quickly. I had lots of medication to take beforehand. The Valium I took an hour before I was due to start chemo took away all of my worries and fears. I walked in to the cancer centre and into the chemo rooms without a worry in the world. I also had to start a three day course of emend (aprepitant). One capsule an hour before and another tablet on day two and day three. Another drug I had to take with me, Aloxi, would be inserted into the drip.

Emend (Aprepitant) -*Emend blocks the actions of*

chemicals in the body that trigger nausea and vomiting. Emend is used together with other medications to prevent nausea and vomiting that may be caused by surgery or cancer chemotherapy. It is given ahead of time and will not treat nausea or vomiting that you already have.

Dexamethasone - *Treating certain conditions associated with decreased adrenal gland function. It is also used to treat severe inflammation due to certain conditions, including severe asthma, severe allergies, rheumatoid arthritis, ulcerative colitis, certain blood disorders, lupus, multiple sclerosis, and certain eye and skin conditions. It may also be used for other conditions as determined by your doctor. Dexamethasone tablets is a corticosteroid. It works by decreasing or preventing tissues from responding to inflammation. It also modifies the body's response to certain immune stimulation.*

Valium (Diazepam) - *Diazepam belongs to a group of medicines called benzodiazepines. Diazepam helps in the treatment of anxiety, muscle spasms and convulsions.*

As usual, Jonathan was by my side. He came with me to chemo just like he had to almost every appointment. Without him I would have gone through it all alone. He had taken more time off work but would be returning in a little over a week. Money was very tight at that time because Jonathan was down as a casual, although he worked full time, so any time off was without pay. We were lucky that he had a great, understanding employer who had allowed him so much time off.

Friday 19th April, at 11am was my first chemo. We had to stop at reception of the cancer centre first and then go around to the chemo rooms. At the chemo rooms we had to wait until the nurses were ready for us. It was going to be a long day.

The chemo room was quite large with about eight very large electronic comfy leather chairs for patients to relax in and chairs for visitors. Soft music played in the background. As we walked in every patient and visitor watched us. I was by far the youngest patient there and that always surprises me. Some people were obviously having their first chemo and others looked like they were having their second or even last chemotherapy. I took a seat where we were directed, at the back of the room, with a full view of everything. The chairs were like lounge chairs, they were so comfortable and could be reclined if wanted.

There were about six nurses there and they were all extremely busy, Friday being their busiest day. They were the most caring and friendly nurses I have ever met. Every one of them made me feel like a person, they were gentle, explained what they would be doing and kept checking on me all day. They always have a smile on their faces. They were happy to chat with all the patients and visitors and made sure everyone was comfortable and relaxed. Since then, I have gotten to know them quite well as I go there every month for treatment.

My nurse for the day was Rose, she was responsible for giving me the chemo and looking after me. Rose called for the doctor to check me over due to my cold and chest infection, she decided I would be fine to go ahead with chemo today. Rose first inserted the cannula into my left hand. I was then hooked up to a drip of the first bag of chemo, which included the extra nausea medication. This would be started slowly and quicken up as it went through my veins. The first drip would take almost three hours. I had to put my gloves on and place my hands inside ice packs. I was supposed to leave my hands in there for the whole three hours but it was too cold and I wasn't able to do anything but sit and think, so within an hour my hands were out of the ice and I had removed the gloves. My hands were freezing and I decided to take the chance on getting black nails or for my finger nails to fall off.

Jonathan and I played games on the iPad and our phones, we read the newspaper. I also had a book to read but it was impossible to concentrate. Most of the day was spent watching people or chatting with the nurses and some patients. We were given lunch and Jonathan went for a walk.

When the first bag of chemo had finished the second bag was hooked up. This was going to be quicker than the first, only taking about two hours. Mine wasn't the longest, some patients' chemo would take eight hours and others had to come in and have it every day.

I was fairly relaxed whilst having the chemo run into

me, as relaxed as you can possibly be anyway. I couldn't concentrate on anything for too long and the day seemed to drag on but we were all made to feel comfortable by the nurses, we were looked after well.

When both drips had finally been emptied most of the people had already gone home. It was late afternoon. I was unhooked from the drip and the cannula removed. I was finally able to go home. I felt tired and a little weak but otherwise I felt fine. I had a list to read over when I got home and directions to follow. Jonathan drove us home and I curled up in bed to rest.

Some of the main instructions to follow were:
Take medications as prescribed
Flush the toilet twice on full flush with the seat down and wash hands thoroughly. Small amounts of chemotherapy stays in your system for up to seven days after treatment.
Take your temperature every morning and night. Immediately contact your nurse or doctor if you develop a fever of 38c or more, or if you develop any signs or symptoms of infection.
If you develop any unexpected or severe side effects, you must also contact the cancer centre staff and/or attend emergency. You develop a rash or other allergic reaction such as swollen eye lids, lips, hands or feet, or experience problems breathing. You have severe uncontrolled nausea or vomiting. You develop uncontrolled diarrhoea. You have bleeding or bruising. You develop pain at the injection site.

Report to the treatment team if you develop a sore throat/mouth or mouth ulcers.
You get constipation.
You develop tingling or pins and needles in hands or feet.
You experience flu-like symptoms and/or pains in joints.
You develop any other side effects.

Other instructions were-
For two days after treatment drink at least 8 to 10 glasses of fluid and empty your bladder frequently. Rinse your mouth after each meal and before going to bed with salty water or bicarbonate mouthwash.

I would be most at risk of getting an infection 10 to 14 days after having chemotherapy. I was advised, during that time, to avoid contact with sick people and minimise time spent in crowded places. It would be best to stay home and have minimal visitors. Most importantly, if I became unwell, developed chills, developed a temperature above 38c or felt short of breath to go to my nearest hospital emergency immediately.

There was so much information, it was scary that so many things could happen. I read through the possible side effects and hoped I wouldn't get many of them. Some were immediate and for other side effects the onset could be days or weeks. Some of those were-

Immediate (hours – days)
Allergic Reaction – skin rash, itching, fever, pain, dizziness, wheezing and shortness of breath. Contact nurse immediately.
Nausea and Vomiting - If you feel unwell or vomit tell your doctor or nurse.
Changes in Sense of smell and taste – Changes in taste and smell are common. Food may become bland or taste metallic. Eat sugar free mints or chew gum. Marinate meats in juice or wine, flavour food with sauces.

Onset Days to Weeks

Increased Risk of Infection – Neutropenia is when white blood cells, called neutrophils are low. Neutrophils are a type of white blood cell that helps fight infection. If you develop a fever 38c or higher, have shivers or feel unwell, call an ambulance to take you to the nearest hospital emergency. Do not delay as this is life-threatening.

Low Red Blood Cell Count – A low red blood cell count can cause you to feel more tired than usual. You may feel light-headed, dizzy and appear pale. Tell your nurse as you may need a blood transfusion. If you become short of breath, develop chest pain or an irregular heartbeat, go straight to the hospital emergency.

Sore Mouth – Tell your nurse if you develop a sore mouth, pain on swallowing or a white coating on your tongue.

Hair Loss – May start within a few weeks of beginning treatment. It can occur on all parts of the body, including eyebrows and eyelashes.

Poor Concentration – Memory changes and being unable to concentrate are common but generally improve once treatment has completed.

Nail Damage – Your nails may grow more slowly, become darker, develop ridges or white lines and become brittle and flaky. In some cases you may lose your nails completely.

Menopausal Symptoms – You may have irregular or no menstrual periods, vaginal dryness, hot flashes, sweating, mood swings, or problems sleeping.

 The list goes on but they were the main and most concerning side effects. I was hoping for the minimum and I followed my instructions carefully and thoroughly but I was to get most of those side effects, within the first 8 days.

After returning home post chemo I remember feeling well but waiting for it to hit me. For the first three days I was feeling quite normal. No signs of any side effects at all and I remember telling everyone how good I felt and if this is how I will feel through all of it then I'm happy to continue having chemotherapy. I was surprised and happy about how I was feeling. I followed my instructions exactly and drank more than enough water and rinsed my mouth after every meal. I was elated that I was still able to eat properly. My medication for nausea and the dexamethasone was only to be taken for the first three days. I thought at the time that was because they were the worse days for nausea and once I passed those days I would be fine. I was very wrong.

As soon as the first three days were over and I stopped with the extra medication I started feeling sick. Day four I was feeling nauseas. I couldn't eat and could only manage to drink water. Everything smelt and tasted disgusting to me. Foods and drinks tasted bland and I had the well-known metallic taste in my mouth. I was feeling very lethargic and spent most of my time on the lounge or in bed. I had pain all over my body and a shocking headache. I couldn't have anything but water. I only had maxalon left to take for nausea and that didn't help at all. By that night diarrhoea had set in and I couldn't keep anything down, not even water. The gastro medication wasn't working. I was doubled over in pain in my chest and stomach. My chesty cough had gotten considerably worse and I was struggling to breathe. Jonathan called an ambulance that night and I was taken to the hospital emergency department. I had a chest x-ray and ultrasound, blood and urine tests were also taken. I was dehydrated, although I had kept up with the water, and I was put on a drip of fluids. I was told my blood work was ok, my white cells hadn't dropped too low. Once the drip had finished, I again felt more like myself. I realised then just how awful I was feeling. It surprised me the difference before and after the drip. My x-ray showed the start of pneumonia. I was put on a drip of antibiotics. I couldn't wait to get back home again, once the drips had finished. The doctor had been in to see me a few times. I had to stay in emergency overnight for observation but luckily for me, the next morning, the doctor gave me the option of staying in the hospital for a few days or going home. Of course I chose to go home. I was so happy that they allowed it because I really didn't want to stay, once I was feeling better.

I was reasonably well for the next two days. By Friday, Jonathan had called the hospital and spoke to the nurse who told us to come in for a check-up. Again, I wasn't able to hold anything down and I was feeling extremely lethargic. At the hospital, cancer centre, I was given a blood test and two drips of fluids. Dr. Hay came in to see me and gave me extra nausea medication and pain relief. My blood test results returned with a very low white blood cell count. I was told I wasn't neutropenic, at this stage, but I was at risk. Dr. Hay asked me if I wanted to stay in the hospital, for observation, over the weekend, but she also gave me the option of going home. I chose to go home. After the second drip of fluids had gone though I was feeling really well again. I had medication that would help me with nausea, so I was confident that I would feel better at home. One of the chemo nurses explained to me what neutropenia was and the importance of taking my temperature regularly. She told me the minute my temperature rises above 38c it is extremely important to get to hospital as soon as possible. She told me that she knows of a few people who died because they were neutropenic and didn't seek medical attention quickly enough. That put the fear of god into me. I'm still not sure if I needed to hear that but it did make me take this very seriously and pay close attention to my temperature. I was told to avoid going out or having visitors over the next week as any germ going around I would easily catch and my body wouldn't be able to fight it.

We left the cancer centre and returned home, confident that I would feel better now that I had extra nausea medications and also nervous about my white cell count being so low.

Neutropenia

Neutropenia is a low level of neutrophils, a type of white blood cell. All white blood cells help the body fight infection. Neutrophils fight infection by destroying harmful bacteria and fungi or yeast that invade the body. Neutrophils are made in the bone marrow. Bone marrow is the spongy tissue found inside larger bones such as the pelvis, vertebrae, and ribs.

Some level of neutropenia occurs in about half of people with cancer who are receiving chemotherapy. It is a common side effect in people with leukemia. If you have neutropenia, pay close attention to personal hygiene, such as hand washing, to lower your risk of infection.

People who have neutropenia have a higher risk of developing serious infections. This is because they do not have enough neutrophils to destroy organisms that cause infection. People with severe or long-lasting neutropenia are more likely to develop an infection.

Signs and symptoms of neutropenia

Neutropenia itself may not cause any symptoms. Patients usually find out they have neutropenia from a blood test or when an infection develops. Some people will feel more fatigued when they have neutropenia. Your doctor will schedule regular blood tests to look for neutropenia and other blood-related side effects of chemotherapy.

For patients with neutropenia, even a minor infection can quickly become serious. Talk with your doctor right away if you experience any of the following signs of infection:

- A fever, which is a temperature of 100.5°F or higher
- Chills or sweating
- Sore throat, sores in the mouth, or a toothache
- Abdominal pain
- Pain near the anus
- Pain or burning when urinating, or urinating often
- Diarrhea or sores around the anus
- A cough or shortness of breath
- Any redness, swelling, or pain, particularly around a cut, wound, or where a catheter was placed
- Unusual vaginal discharge or itching

Managing and treating neutropenia

When neutrophil levels begin to drop depends on the type or dose of chemotherapy. Neutrophil counts generally start to drop about a week after each round of chemotherapy begins. Neutrophil levels reach a low point called the nadir about 7 to 14 days after treatment. At this point, you are most likely to develop an infection. Your neutrophil count then starts to rise again as your bone marrow resumes normal production of neutrophils. However, it may take three to four weeks to reach a normal level again.

When your neutrophil level returns to normal, your body is ready for the next round of chemotherapy. Your doctor may delay the next round of chemotherapy or lower the dose for the following reasons:

- You develop neutropenia
- Your neutrophil level does not return to normal quickly enough

Your doctor may recommend antibiotics during periods of prolonged neutropenia to try to prevent infections from occurring.

If chemotherapy causes neutropenia with a fever, your doctor may prescribe medications called white blood cell growth factors. These drugs help the body make more white blood cells.

Source – cancer.net

Saturday was day 8 since I had chemo. Jonathan had taken leave from work and was due to return the next day, Sunday. He had an early start and had to be up by 5am. For all the reading I had done about chemo and the side effects, we thought I would be feeling better by then and would be on the way up. We were wrong!

We stayed home all of Saturday, the words from the nurse the day before still fresh in my mind. I started by taking my temperature every hour and it was always normal. I was taking my medications as prescribed and I was feeling quite good. As the day went on I checked my temperature less often. By early in the evening, after dinner, I was feeling a little strange. Not unwell exactly, no headaches or other side effects, just an odd feeling.

I went to the bathroom and started vomiting and had diarrhoea. It was the worst case I ever had. It scared me because it was so violent and unexpected. I was sweating and shaking. I couldn't stand straight and the room was spinning. I was stuck in the bathroom for half an hour.

When I was able to return to my bed, I remembered I hadn't checked my temperature for a couple of hours. I heard the fast beeping first, so I knew my temperature was up but when I looked it was on 39c. I immediately panicked and called for Jonathan. He ran into the room and I told him my temperature was up. Within seconds he was on the phone to 000 emergency. He relayed instructions to me of what to do. The operator told me to lay down on my bed. I continued taking my temperature and it kept rising. It was now 41c.

For whatever reasons Jonathan was transferred to a doctor and then another doctor and back to 000. He seemed to be on the phone forever and not really getting anywhere. Finally, for what seemed like an hour later but was probably only ten minutes, a paramedic arrived. He was straight into action, all the while talking to me and calming me down, and getting details of what has been happening. He hooked me up to a heart monitor, took my blood pressure and put a cannula in my hand. My heart was racing and my blood pressure was low. He put me on oxygen. The paramedic explained that he had arrived in a car and the ambulance would be here shortly. Apparently, we called 000 just before 7pm which is the changeover time, the start of new shifts, and a difficult time to get an ambulance. The paramedic explained to me the importance of being seen to quickly once I get to hospital. He told me not to wait any longer than one hour to have an i.v of antibiotics. He told me to make a fuss if I haven't been seen to and treated. It was extremely important for my health and my own life that I take control and demand what I need, if necessary. Waiting could result in a much more serious case or even death. The paramedic's words scared me but also made me understand how serious this was. I have never forgotten what he said to me that night, I am so grateful to him, because had he not taken the time and explained to me what I had to do, maybe things could have been worse. He was the second person to tell me how important it was to get medical attention quickly, so I knew now just how serious this was.

Two ambulances arrived a short time later. The paramedic explained the situation to them.

My poor little girl, Annabelle, was in the lounge room all this time, crying and panicking. My heart broke for her, she was scared and worried about what was going on. As soon as I was alert enough I asked where she was, she had been in the lounge room by herself this whole time. Annabelle was still not yet six years old. I wish she had never had to see any of this. The paramedic was fantastic with her, telling her that Mummy was a bit sick but will go to hospital to get better. He even showed her all of his gadgets and the monitor explaining to her in childlike terms what they are for. He calmed her down, thank goodness.

A short time later I was walked out of the house to the ambulance. I tried to comfort Annabelle on my way out and tell her I was ok. Jonathan and Annabelle were going to follow behind the ambulance to the hospital. I knew this time that I would be staying in hospital and wouldn't be lucky enough to return home so soon.

We arrived at the hospital and I was taken straight to a bed after seeing the triage nurse. My temperature remained at 43c. I was given a hospital mask to wear, to protect me from any germs in the hospital. I was very thin and had my funky hairstyle at the time, so I imagine other patients in emergency were staring at me because they thought I was a drug addict or that I was contagious. It made me feel uncomfortable. I was in emergency because I was very sick, a cancer patient, but the group of people across from me were staring and watching me like I had the plague. I was put into a gown and I was placed on a drip of fluids and given Panadol to try to reduce my temperature and help with the headache I had developed. I asked about antibiotics but I was told I had to wait to see the doctor. My oncologist had also been contacted. Jonathan and Annabelle arrived and I asked them to help me to the bathroom because I had to give a urine sample. I was slow and unsteady on my feet. To prove I wasn't just being paranoid, as I walked near the group of people who continued to stare and give me dirty looks, they quickly moved to the other side of the bed of the person they were visiting. We didn't say anything to them, we ignored them, and continued to the toilets. It upset me and made me feel self- conscious but people like that are not worth words.

The on duty doctor was quick to see me, within the hour of arriving. He asked lots of questions about my cancer and treatment. He took blood for a blood test. I told him I needed antibiotics and quickly but he told me they were waiting to hear from my oncologist for instructions. Every ten minutes I was having my temperature and blood pressure taken. I was starting to panic about not having any antibiotics yet.

The people opposite me obviously overheard the conversation with the doctor. Suddenly, they were smiling at us and looking at us with sympathy. One of them actually came over to my cubicle and offered Jonathan a chair. I was upset at how they had treated me when I arrived in emergency and I still remember today how they made me feel. I tried very hard to not even look in their direction but that was very hard to do, especially since they were watching us closely.

Every time a nurse or doctor came to my cubicle I asked for antibiotics, I was panicking because time was passing and the words of the paramedic stuck in my head. I explained that I was told how important it was for me to get them quickly. It was almost three hours after I arrived in emergency that I was finally hooked up to a drip of antibiotics.

Just as I thought, I wasn't given the option of going home this time. I was just too sick. Jonathan had work early the next morning and it was now getting late. I was waiting to be moved to a room in a ward. I would be staying in hospital. Jonathan stayed with me until I was moved to a ward, that wasn't until almost one in the morning.

I was moved into a single room. My temperature was still around 41c. By morning I was moved to a different room, opposite the nurses' desk. I was told because I was neutropenic the door would remain closed and anybody entering would have to wear a gown and mask. There was a sign placed on my door warning people of infection control. I guess some people might have thought that I had something contagious, rather than I was the one in danger of contracting any infections. My meals were usually left outside the room. I wasn't allowed out of the room, so unless a nurse bought my meals into me I didn't get them. I wasn't really eating anything anyway as I still couldn't hold anything down. Most of the time I slept. I would usually only wake when

I was disturbed by the doctors or nurses changing my drip. I stayed on the antibiotics and was actually having two different types intravenously.

I remained in there for four nights. Jonathan was back at work so I hardly saw him and Annabelle, only for up to half an hour at night. My sister, Georgie, was taking care of Annabelle everyday whilst Jonathan was at work until he had a day off mid-week. Jonathan picked her up every night and took her home. Friends from school came and picked up Annabelle and took her to school. My mother-in-law came and visited me twice and stayed for hours, just sitting by my bed knitting, most of the time I was sleeping, I just wasn't able to keep my eyes open. These people all made a difference and they will never know how grateful I was to them.

I was taken to have lots of tests done – CT scans and x-rays. I had to drink a horrible liquid before one of the scans which was very hard to keep down. After that scan I was vomiting violently and had severe diarrhoea. I was stuck in the bathroom, not having enough strength to open the door and return to bed. I was crying and got myself in a real emotional mess. I had to press the emergency buzzer for the nurses to come in and help me back to bed. I was taking so much medication to stop the diarrhoea and vomiting but nothing could stop it. I was exhausted.

I had so many blood tests, about four each day that I had to start having blood taken from my feet and legs. Nurses checked my temperature two or three times each time because they thought the reading was incorrect, my temperature remained high between 40c and 42c. Yet another unwanted side effect from chemo, I was also diagnosed with ulcerative colitis. The reason for the severe diarrhoea.

Ulcerative Colitis is a disease that is characterized by inflammation and micro-ulcers in the superficial layers of the large intestine. The inflammation usually occurs in the rectum and lower part of the colon, but it may affect the entire large intestine (pan colitis). Ulcerative colitis can very rarely affect the small intestine in its distal portion (Backwash Ileitis).

The inflammation is accompanied usually with diarrhea, which may be profuse and bloody. Micro-ulcers form in places where inflammation has destroyed the cells lining the bowel and these areas bleed and produce pus and mucus. Ulcerative colitis, especially when mild, can be difficult to diagnose because symptoms are similar to other intestinal disorders, most notably the other type of IBD called Crohn's disease and also irritable bowel syndrome.

Common symptoms of ulcerative colitis include:

- abdominal pain
- increased abdominal sounds
- bloody stools
- diarrhea
- fever
- rectal pain

- weight loss
- malnutrition
- joint pain
- joint swelling
- nausea
- vomiting
- skin ulcers
- mouth sores

By Wednesday, I woke in the morning feeling so much better. My temperature had dropped back to normal the day before and I was no longer so sick. I was able to get out of bed and sit in the chair. I was still dosing on and off but not nearly as much as I had been. I felt like I had come back to life again. One of the nurses came in in the morning and told me I would be going home today after I saw my oncologist. I was so excited, I was ready to go home. Now that I was feeling better I was bored in hospital and needed to get home to my family. I sat, waiting all day for a doctor to come in and see me. I even started asking the nurses if my doctor was here. No-one turned up to see me. I was so disappointed and upset because I had my hopes up to go home. By early evening I asked another nurse why my doctor hadn't been in and I told her that the morning nurses had told me I would be going home. I was anxious by then, I always get that way in hospital. Once I'm feeling better I just want to get out of there. That lovely nurse, knowing I desperately wanted to go home, called my doctor in to see me. By the time the doctor came in it was after seven at night. She checked me over and was talking about giving me more antibiotics and blood tests. I told her I wanted to go home. I couldn't stay any longer now that I was feeling better. She didn't agree that I was ready but did call my oncologist who said if my last blood results came back with my white cell count above 1 then I could go home that night. My results were 1.1. I was so lucky and felt so relieved and happy. Four nights had been more than long enough to be in hospital. I was given scripts for antibiotics and nausea medication as well as pain relief. Within the hour I was wheeled down to the exit and on my way home.

Recovery

I was on a long road to recovery after that incident. I still often tell people that chemo almost killed me. The doctors explain it as being that my body couldn't tolerate chemo. I decided, with the backing of my oncologist, that I would not be having anymore cycles of chemotherapy. I couldn't take the chance again that something like that would happen. A few days after returning home, one of Dr. Hay's registrars who I had seen in hospital several times, called me. She was checking on my progress but also wanted to ask me if I would consider a different type of chemo, one that is not as strong as the first one that I was on. My immediate answer was no. I didn't need any time to think about it and no-one was going to talk me into it this time. A.C was the chemotherapy she wanted me to try, she said it was less toxic and not as strong as the one I was given. My reply to that was, why wasn't I given that in the first place then? Why was I given the strongest chemo? But I didn't get any answers to my questions.

For weeks after coming home from hospital I had doctors' appointments galore. My blood was checked regularly and my white cells remained low. A few times I was doubled over with pain due to the newly diagnosed colitis. I remained on antibiotics for several weeks.

Once I was stronger, I saw Dr. Hay in her rooms at the cancer centre. Arrangements were made for me to see the radiation oncologist, Dr. Brown and to begin radiation. I was given a script for tamoxifen to begin once I finished radiation. Since I didn't finish chemotherapy I was also offered another, alternative treatment of Goseralin. Also known as Zoladex Implants. I would have the injections every four weeks for either two or five years. Zoladex injections would close down my ovaries. Combined with tamoxifen I was given an excellent chance of staying cancer free.

Over the weeks I got stronger and felt more like myself. Once the effects of chemo wore off. I suffered strongly with chemo brain and still do. I could be mid-sentence in conversation and totally forget what I was saying. I forget a lot of things from my age to where I am going or what I was about to do. So far though, I haven't forgotten where I live, so that is a good thing.

My white blood cell count is often low, even two years down the track. Chemo and the side effects have hung around for a long time. I only had one cycle, I can't imagine what my life would be like now if I had completed chemo.

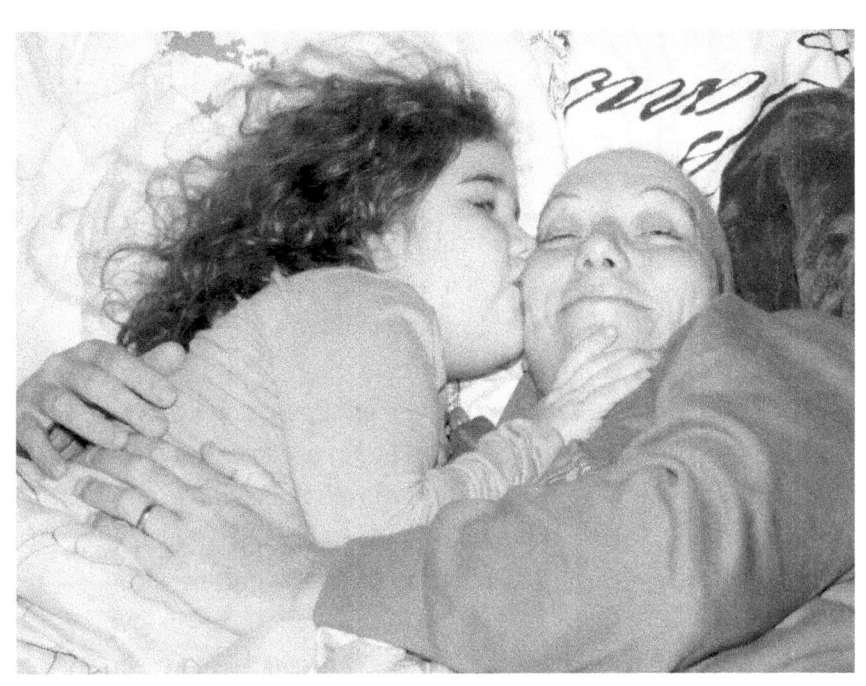

Radiotherapy

My first appointment with Dr. Brown was at the end of April. Yet another lovely female doctor. My hospital doesn't offer radiotherapy so I will have to attend the next closest hospital in my area. Arrangements were made that I would go to the cancer centre and be scanned and tattooed ready to begin radiotherapy. My appointment wasn't for another two weeks and it would be a further two weeks before I actually started radiation. Dr. Brown went through all the details with me.

I would have radiation every day for eight weeks. Nine day fortnights because on the tenth day the machines are serviced. The actual treatment only lasts less than five minutes each time. By week three I should expect to start seeing red burns across my chest. These may blister and then I will have to seek treatment from the nurses. I was told to use sorbolene cream daily to help moisturise the skin.

Dr Brown explained to me what the side effects of radiotherapy are, and although I may not get them all, it is important to know beforehand.

Radiotherapy works by killing any cancer cells that may be present in the breast following surgery. The normal cells are also affected. Some side effects will occur early, within days to weeks of starting treatment. Other side effects may develop in the 'long term', months to years after completing treatment.

Common Side Effects -

Tiredness

Skin reddening and irritation

Breast swelling

Occasional aches and pains in the breast

Breast firmness, scarring and skin pigmentation

Temporary(sometimes permanent) loss of armpit hair

Sore throat

Uncommon Side Effects-

Lung inflammation and scarring. A small amount of lung will be included in the treatment beam. Some lung scarring can occur which may show in x-rays months to years later. A small number of patients, 1 in 100, may develop lung inflammation.

Rib pain and fracture. Some patients will complain of rib pain and tenderness some months or years after treatment. Approximately, 1 -2 in 100 may have a rib fracture due to weakening of the rib bone.

Lymphedema. This can result from having treatment in the arm pit area. The risk may be between 9 – 15 patients in every 100. If the lymph nodes area is treated.

Nausea. Is very uncommon.

Rare Side Effects-
Heart damage
Secondary malignancy
Severe breast hardness and shrinkage
Damage to the nerves which supply the arm.

Radiotherapy Planning

My first visit for radiotherapy was for planning. I had to be marked up for the start of radiotherapy. It involved a 5 – 10 minute meeting with a nurse to discuss what would be happening today. I would have a CT scan and be placed in exactly the same position that I will need to be in for treatment. Measurements will be taken and I will have three small, permanent tattoos. The tattoos will assist staff when getting me in to the correct position. Planning took approximately two hours. I still remember getting the tattoos, one in the middle of my chest and one on each side of my body. The tattoos are tiny, like a freckle, but I remember thinking that they hurt and it turned me off getting any real tattoos, for the time being anyway.

Treatment

I started treatment two weeks after planning. It was mid-May, 2013. I had a twenty – thirty minute drive each way, every day. Some days Jonathan was able to come with me, but mostly I went alone. Radiation was so much easier than chemo. The hardest part for me was the drive there and back every day. Every day, two hours after treatment, I would get extremely tired and have to take a nap or at least have a lay down. I was lucky that my appointments were always made during school times, so I was able to have my treatment and return in time to pick up Annabelle from school. There was however one time when Annabelle was unwell and I had no one to take care of her, so I had no choice but to take her with me. She wasn't able to come in the room with me, due to the dangers of radiation, so I had to leave her in the waiting room by herself. She had just turned six. That was the hardest moment of my life and I panicked the whole time I was having treatment. I couldn't wait to get back out to Annabelle. I had a fear that she may not be there when I came out. Although, I told her not to talk to anyone and not to move from her seat and I left her playing with her iPad, I was worried about her sitting out there by herself. When treatment was finished I almost ran out of the room, fearing that Annabelle was gone but she was still sitting there where I had left her. She told me later that she had cried when I was gone because she was scared by herself.

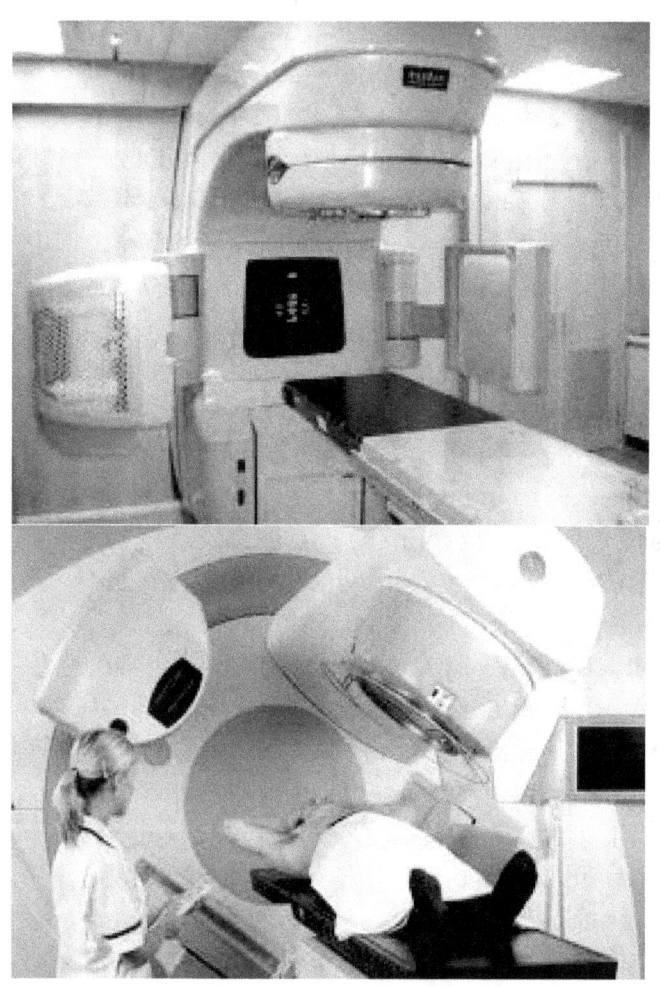

Most days I was in and out within an hour. The treatment itself only took about ten minutes. Sometimes there were delays with machines or a backlog of patients waiting for treatment, but mostly it was over with quickly. The therapists were all lovely and caring. I would report to the desk every day and then wait in the waiting room until my name was called. I had my own pigeon hole where my gown and a basket for my clothing were kept. Each day, I would be called by a therapist, change in to my gown and begin radiation. The longest part was making sure I was in the correct position and the same areas receive radiation.

At first, I did feel a little anxious and it took me a couple of weeks to get used to it. The machine would move very close to my body and face. It was always over with quickly though and there was soft music playing in the background.

Once every two weeks I would see Dr. Brown so she could check my burns and how I was going. The visits were short but comforting, knowing that I was doing well.

By week three my breast area started turning red, like a sunburn. I was using the sorbolene cream as directed. So far that was my only side effect besides of course being tired every day.

As the weeks went on my skin was turning a darker red and becoming itchy. By my second last week of therapy I started developing blisters in the areas where I was receiving radiation. Under my breast mainly and near my underarm area. The therapists on my machine noticed and sent me to see the nurses after my treatment. I was given gels and creams to use every day and my blistered areas were treated and bandaged. I had to change the dressing daily and return to the nurses every three days to be checked. Eventually, the blisters broke and once I was finished with my treatment I began to heal.

It was such a relief when I finished treatment. I was so happy that I had completed it. Not having to drive to the hospital every day was a great feeling. I still became tired every day at about the same time, for the next few months.

I didn't need to see Dr. Brown again for six months.

Hormonal Therapies

Once I had completed radiotherapy it was time to start with the hormonal therapy. My cancer was er+ and pr+ therefore my treatment would be tamoxifen for ten years and goserelin implants (zoladex) for two – five years.

Tamoxifen and Zoladex are hormonal therapy medicines used to lower the risk of breast cancer coming back (recurrence) in premenopausal women diagnosed with early-stage, hormone-receptor-positive breast cancer.
Estrogen can make hormone-receptor-positive breast cancers grow. Hormonal therapy medicines treat hormone-receptor-positive breast cancers in two ways:

- by blocking the action of estrogen in the body
- by lowering the amount of estrogen in the body

At the time, having both tamoxifen and zoladex, my doctors and I were all confident that my cancer would not return. I believed, wrongly, that it was near impossible to get hormonal positive cancer again. I was confident that my cancer had been removed and this treatment would stop any future cancer.
My life was never going to be the same again. Once I started this treatment it was goodbye forever to the old me, the pre-cancer me. This treatment was going to put

me into menopause and would age my body significantly. I would also gain an enormous amount of weight.

Tamoxifen. What is it and what does it do.

Often referred to by pink sisters (women diagnosed with breast cancer), as tamoxabitch. The side effects can be nasty and will put you into menopause. Roll on hot flushes and sweats. A very common side effect is weight gain. At my lowest weight, at the start of this journey when I was having chemo, I dropped down to a very low 67kg. My lowest weight since I was a teenager. At a height of 5' 11", and weighing just sixty seven kilos, I was quite thin and sickly looking. Two years into taking tamoxifen I have gained 50kgs and now weigh a massive 117kgs. My regular weight, pre-cancer was around 80 kgs. I am now wearing a size 20 in clothing. The biggest I have ever been and the most I have ever weighed. No amount of exercise or change of diet helps. I have not been able to shift the weight whatsoever. I usually make a joke of my weight and the size I am now wearing, but now that doctors have started telling me to lose weight, I am getting a little concerned about it, especially if I continue to gain weight.

Tamoxifen blocks the effects of estrogen — a reproductive hormone that influences the growth and development of many breast tumours. Tamoxifen belongs to a class of drugs known as selective estrogen receptor modulators (SERMs), and it reduces the effects of estrogen in most areas of the body, including the breast. In the uterus, tamoxifen acts like an estrogen and encourages the growth of the lining of the uterus.

Tamoxifen is prescribed as a pill you take once a day by mouth. For breast cancer risk reduction, tamoxifen is typically taken for a total of five years. The risk reduction benefit continues for 10 years after you stop taking tamoxifen.

Common side effects

The most common side effects that people have when taking tamoxifen are menopausal symptoms. These include:

- hot flushes
- night sweats and sleep disturbance
- vaginal irritation (such as dryness and itching)
- loss of sex drive (libido)
- mood changes.

Women who are still having regular periods may find that these change. For example, they may be lighter and/or irregular or may stop altogether. Vaginal discharge is common when taking tamoxifen.

If you are post-menopausal, tamoxifen slows down the process of bone loss, reducing the risk of osteoporosis (thinning of the bones). However, pre-menopausal women may be at risk of thinning of the bones when taking tamoxifen. This is unlikely to lead to osteoporosis unless treatment has been given to stop the ovaries from working as well.

Taking tamoxifen increases the risk of blood clots such as deep vein thrombosis (DVT). People with a DVT are at risk of developing a pulmonary embolism. This is when part of the blood clot breaks away and travels to the lung.

Tamoxifen can also affect the lining of the uterus or womb (known as the endometrium), which may become thickened. Occasionally tamoxifen may cause polyps or ovarian cysts or very rarely, cancer of the uterus (womb).

Tamoxifen can occasionally cause changes to how the liver works. These changes are usually very mild and unlikely to cause any symptoms. Once you finish your treatment your liver will almost certainly go back to normal.

Other side effects

- eyesight problems
- hair thinning/hair loss
- increase in downy facial hair
- weight gain
- joint pains
- tiredness
- headaches

While you are taking tamoxifen you will be advised not to get pregnant as it may harm a developing baby. Even if your periods stop while you are taking tamoxifen you could still get pregnant.

The risk of uterine cancer for premenopausal women taking tamoxifen is very low, compared with those who have undergone menopause. The benefits of tamoxifen outweigh the risks in premenopausal women who have an increased risk of breast cancer due to a strong family history of the disease or a personal history of precancerous breast changes.

Tamoxifen works on the whole body (known as systemic treatment) and blocks the effects of estrogen on the receptors. This helps to stop any breast cancer cells from growing.

I started on a 20mg dose of tamoxifen mid-August. I had put off taking it for as long as possible. I was a little concerned about the side effects, I found the information about most side effects by going online. My oncologist, Dr, Hay was still seeing me every month at this stage.

Within days of starting tamoxifen I started getting debilitating headaches. Most of the time I wasn't able to even get out of bed. No amount of pain medication worked to stop them only to relieve them slightly. I saw my g.p because the headaches continued, he sent me immediately for a CT scan on my head, to rule out a brain tumor and also sent me to get my eyes checked. Both came back clear. My doctor suggested I see Dr. Hay as it could be a side effect of tamoxifen. I stopped tamoxifen after a week, the headaches continued for several more days. I saw Dr. Hay and explained to her that I had stopped taking tamoxifen due to the headaches. Dr Hay suggested I stop tamoxifen for a month and then restart with a 10mg dose for a further month before going back to a 20mg dose. By October, I was back taking tamoxifen at a lower dose. There were no headaches and no signs of any real side effects that I noticed, but once I boosted my dose to 20mg the side effects were obvious and very real.

During chemo and for a while afterwards I was having hot flushes. They finally stopped whilst I was having radiation. Once I started tamoxifen again and combined with the zoladex injections, they came back with a vengeance. Out of the blue I would start sweating so badly that it looked like I had just had a shower, combined with nausea, they are not fun at all. I feel like I am burning up from head to toe. The heat overpowers me and I feel like I am on fire. I feel embarrassed to be near people. My hot flushes are every ten to fifteen minutes and I have no control whatsoever over them. During the warmer weather they seem so much worse and the moment I lay down in bed I will get a hot flush. I can go from freezing to boiling in an instant. I will put on a jacket or jumper and within minutes have to strip off because I am overheating. Dr. Hay suggested a natural treatment that I could try which may help with menopausal symptoms – being my hot flushes. It was available at a pharmacy and called black cohosh. I tried it for a few weeks but it didn't help at all.

I continued on with tamoxifen for the next two years. My hot flushes continue and my weight gain excessive. I thought they were the only side effects until recently I started getting lower pelvic pain. A pelvic ultrasound showed I had a cyst in the endometrium caused by tamoxifen. My doctors were not concerned and let it go for three months when I was sent for another ultrasound. This time it showed that I have developed three cysts. Still, none of my doctors are concerned by this as the report states they were caused by tamoxifen. I don't know if I should be concerned or not about this, if it's possible that those will turn cancerous or not but my doctors at the moment are happy to just keep check on them.

Efexor

To assist with my hot flushes I was offered Efexor. Efexor is an anti-depressant but is also widely used to assist breast cancer patients with menopause symptoms. A very low dose is taken to help with the effects of hot flushes. I started on 37.5mg tablets and did get some relief from my hot flushes. They didn't stop completely but they did ease and the sweating was less noticeable. They are not supposed to work as an anti-depressant for me but I think they do to some extent.

Unfortunately, over time my body must get used to them so I have had my dosage put up several times so that now I am on the maximum dose for hot flushes which is 150mg per day. I am at the point now, two years after starting Efexor that my hot flushes and sweats are back to the point of being very strong. I don't think Efexor are working any longer for my hot flushes but do assist with my moods.

Something I have learned by looking online is that Efexor is not easy to stop. I didn't know this when I started taking them and I was never told by my doctors. You have to be weaned off them slowly over a long period of time. Just missing a dose has caused me to feel like I am getting electric shocks run through my body and I find it difficult to get out of bed. I feel that way for days after just being several hours late with a dose. I hate to imagine what happens when you try to stop taking them. Another fear I have about stopping them is, what if they are helping my hot flushes and once I stop taking them my hot flushes get increasingly worse.

Another side effect I have since starting Efexor is hypertension, high blood pressure, and I am now on medication to control it. Weight gain is also another side effect.

Things you must not do

Do not suddenly stop taking Efexor-XR or lower the dose if you have been taking it for some time. If possible, your doctor will gradually reduce the amount you take each day before stopping the medicine completely.

If you stop taking it suddenly, your condition may worsen or you may have unwanted side effects such as:

- Headache
- Nausea and vomiting
- Dizziness
- Insomnia
- Nervousness
- Anxiety
- Confusion and agitation
- Diarrhea

- Sweating
- Loss of appetite
- Tremor
- Flu-like symptoms
- Impaired coordination and balance
- Tingling or numbness of the hands and feet.

Goserelin Implants (Zoladex)

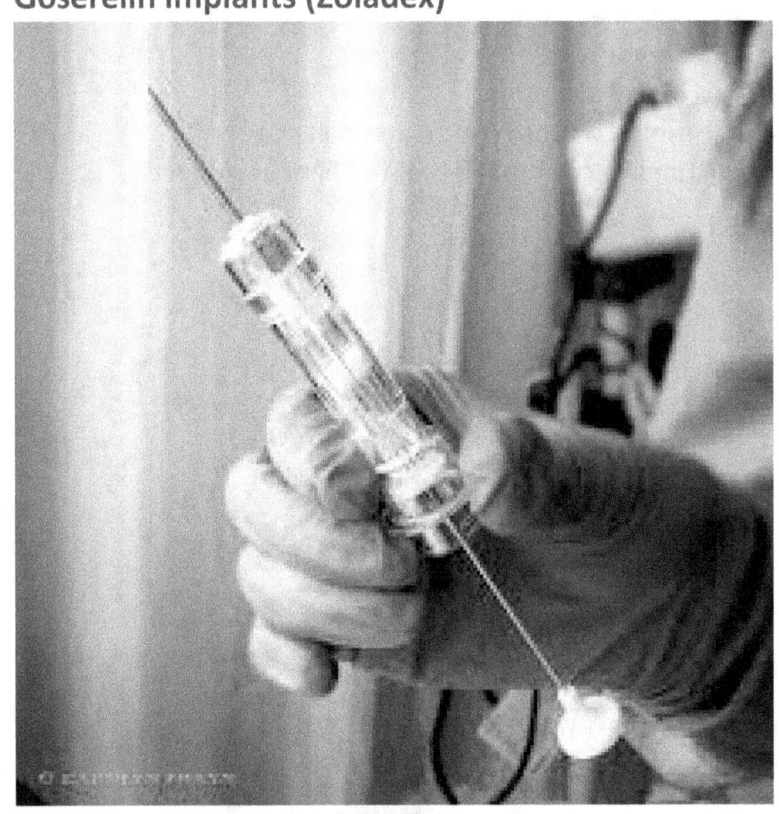

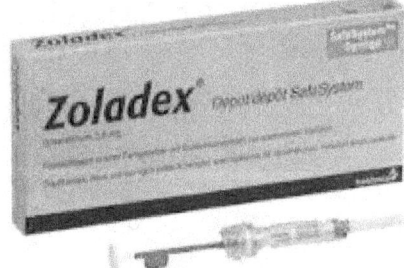

ZOLADEX lowers the amount of sex hormones in the body. In women it reduces the level of oestrogen. In men it reduces the level of testosterone.

ZOLADEX can treat breast cancer in some women before menopause or the 'change of life'. It is not a cure for breast cancer.

ZOLADEX 3.6mg is also used to treat endometriosis and fibroids of the uterus. These are not cancer.

ZOLADEX 3.6mg is used to thin the lining of the womb before surgery.

ZOLADEX 3.6mg is also used in combination with other drugs as part of a treatment for infertility.

ZOLADEX 3.6mg can treat prostate cancer in some men. It is not a cure for prostate cancer.

A ZOLADEX 3.6mg implant will be injected under the skin of your stomach every 28 days.

The implant is a very small pellet that is given by a special needle and syringe known as Safe System. The injection will not hurt very much.

Side Effects

The pellet is designed to slowly release the medicine into your body over four weeks.

- skin rashes
- painful joints
- hot flushes, sweating or feeling faint
- chills
- tingling in fingers or toes
- swelling, soreness or itchiness of the breasts
- vaginal dryness
- headache
- mood changes
- trouble passing urine or experience lower back pain
- your testicles getting smaller

These are all mild side effects of ZOLADEX 3.6mg.

ZOLADEX 3.6mg lowers the amount of sex hormones in your body so your sex drive will probably be reduced.

It is unlikely that you can father a child or fall pregnant while using ZOLADEX 3.6mg, unless it is for infertility treatment.

Most women stop having periods while being treated with ZOLADEX 3.6mg. Some may go through menopause while being given ZOLADEX 3.6mg and not have periods again when the treatment is finished.

In men and in women who have not gone through the 'change of life', ZOLADEX 3.6mg is likely to reduce the amount of calcium in their bones leading to a loss in bone mineral density. It is known that bone mineral density loss partially recovers in the next several months following cessation of therapy. However, doctors do not know if bone mineral density loss will recover completely in every person. Discuss this with your doctor or pharmacist if you are concerned.

If you have a tumour in your pituitary gland, ZOLADEX 3.6mg may make the tumour bleed or collapse. This is very rare but causes severe headaches, sickness, loss of eyesight and unconsciousness.

Every four weeks I go to the cancer centre at the hospital and have my zoladex injection. I've now been having it for two years and am expected to continue for another three years. I have to order the injection in from the pharmacy as no one stocks it as I believe it is too expensive. The full cost of the injection is $335 but I pay $6.10 because I have a health care card. If I had to pay $335 per month then I wouldn't be able to have it as it is too expensive. I get it from the pharmacy and take it to the hospital for a nurse to give me the injection. I have it in my stomach every four weeks. The nurses usually swap sides each injection. Because I have gained weight I have plenty of fat around my stomach that can be pinched and the implant put in, so whilst it is uncomfortable for me it is not usually very painful. The quicker it is done the less painful it is. Sometimes, the nurse has hit a vessel and I have bled a bit and bruised but usually I am fine afterwards. I have been told that ladies who are thin really feel the implant and it is quite painful. Some ladies at the cancer centre have refused to have any more injections of zoladex after a time because it is just too painful for them.

Usually after an injection I feel tired for a few days and my hot flushes worsen by getting stronger for the first week or two. I'm told now that zoladex can cause osteoporosis and I should have had a bone density scan but I haven't as yet. I do get a lot of bone and joint pain between injections but mostly it is manageable with pain medication.

Life goes on

My doctors' appointments continued through 2013 and 2014. Eventually my visits went from monthly to every three months. I continued seeing Dr Hay and Dr Sa. I relied on Dr. Hay for my breast exams, every appointment she would check my breasts for any lumps or signs of change.

My genetics test results came back almost three months after I took the test. Dr Hay called me in to her office and told me that my test results came back positive. I had the BRCA gene. I was surprised by the news but not shocked. It made sense given my family history. Now, I was faced with some big decisions to make. I had to consider having a double mastectomy. That would be the first thing I would have to do. I would also have to tell my sisters who would all now be able to also have the genetics test. I would also have to consider how to tell my distant relatives. I felt obligated to tell them. If I was positive to the gene then Mum was positive to the gene, therefore it was probable that some of her sisters and their children were also positive. Telling them was not a priority though, it was something that I could do later, there were more important things to do right now.

The next day, Dr Tam also called me in to see him. He also had received a copy of my genetics results. He told me that my results had come back and they were "inconclusive". Meaning I don't have the BRCA gene mutation.

My response – What the f***?

I explained to Dr. Tam what had taken place the day before. Dr. Hay told me I was positive for the mutation. I couldn't believe what was happening. One day I have it, the next I don't. Do I have it or not? Who knows?

Dr. Tam printed out his copy and showed me the results. Clearly it stated that I was inconclusive. What does that mean? Dr. Tam wasn't sure either, the report wasn't a very detailed one. I had to wait until the genetics centre called me in to get my results and have them explained to me. The fact that my doctors get them first and can relay the wrong information doesn't sit well with me. I could have reacted differently to finding out I had the gene mutation. How would they know? That is the reason for the counselling, I thought, to explain it to you, in detail and help you through. Otherwise, what is the point of seeing them? I could have just seen my doctors in the first place.

When I had returned from Dr. Tam I had two messages on my phone. One from Dr Hay, apologising that she had given me someone else's genetics results, she didn't actually have mine. Oh my, unbelievable, what a terrible mistake. I was angry about this and planned on telling the genetics councillor if ever I saw her. The second message on my phone was in fact from the genetics centre, they made an appointment for me to go in for my results the following week.

Arriving at the genetics centre I was in a hurry to get this over with. I knew my results were inconclusive already. I now just wanted to know what that meant.

I was told that 'inconclusive' means that I don't have BRCA1 or BRCA2 gene mutations. Good news. BUT, I may have other gene mutations that cannot be tested for at the moment because they don't have enough information. My sisters and other relatives will not be able to have the genetics test, unless they pay thousands of dollars, because I don't have the BRCA1 or BRCA2 gene mutations, therefore they won't have it either. I, being the person in our family with breast cancer, would have to test positive for any of my sisters to be able to test positive.

My reaction to that news. Well no doubt it is a good thing that I don't have the BRCA1 or BRCA2 gene mutations but I was feeling that it had been a whole waste of time. I felt like I was left in limbo, being inconclusive, means I could have another gene mutation but sorry, we can't tell you what that is, because we don't know.

Some people in my circle stopped asking how I was doing after a while. Phone calls or text messages either stopped or were rare. I haven't heard from one of my sisters since I had chemo and I don't have any way of contacting her. I take it in my stride, if people really don't care you can't make them. Life is too short to worry about other people when they can't be bothered even keeping in touch. Instead, I concentrate on the people who do care and the people who have supported me, been by my side, since my diagnosis. The most important people in my life are Jonathan and Annabelle. Everything I do, I do for Annabelle.

We all have our own lives to live and families and responsibilities but it takes only a minute to text someone you care about, a person who you know has been going through a tough time. When a person receives a cancer diagnosis it can change many things in their life, including relationships. I've heard of so many cancer patients losing touch with friends, family or separating from partners once they have been diagnosed with cancer. Some people don't want to or can't see you through treatment, for others they don't know what to say or do. Sadly, many people think once you've had surgery and the cancer has been removed then that is the end of it. Many people don't understand that it is a very long road of treatment. Many of us have to live with the fear of cancer returning every day. The slightest changes in our bodies sends us running back to the doctor in case cancer has returned. For many people they will never be free of cancer and they live everyday hoping it won't be their last.

Once you get that cancer diagnosis, life will never be the same again. Whether your cancer is removed by surgery or not.

For two years following diagnosis of breast cancer I have had my doctors keeping a close eye on me. Every new pain is checked by sending me for tests or scans. I am so grateful to my doctors for always taking notice and listening to me, particularly my local g.p, Dr Tan, who I credit for saving me. I have had so many scans and blood tests over the two year period that I have lost count. My blood tests have always come back with something irregular, usually my white cells are still low and I am usually low in vitamin d and iron. At times I have had to take a daily dose of up to 19 medications. I now also have hypertension (high blood pressure) and I take medication for that too.

Although, life went on, it was a new, different life. Every time there is a new pain I start to worry. I have my yearly mammograms and ultrasounds and I worry about the results. A life after a cancer diagnosis is a life with anxiety. Having so many doctors' appointments and tests and scans gets tiring.

During my routine mammogram and ultrasound in September 2014 my results came back as having a debris filled cyst in my right breast measuring 7mm. It was where my seroma had been after surgery. I rely heavily on my g.p's opinion and he said I would have to see my surgeon Dr. Sa. I would probably have it aspirated. He explained to me that it was obviously filled with something which could be fluid, blood or something else. If Dr Sa again refused to do anything about it then he will send me for a second opinion. I was happy with that because each time I had seen Dr. Sa since my surgery he often brushed things off as being nothing. I still get nervous when I see him since the lecture I received about chemo.

Complex Breast Cysts:
Complex cysts differ from simple cysts in that they have a solid component or debris within the fluid filled sac. They may also have thin walls or septations. They may contain thick fluid, or fluid that contains dead cells. An aspiration is often recommended to make sure it is not solid. Complex breast cysts with an intracystic solid mass have up to 40% incidence of an underlying malignancy. The management of complex breast cysts includes short follow up, needle aspiration or core biopsy and excisional biopsy.

During my visit with Dr. Sa I was nervous about the new cyst in my breast. I expected him to say he would drain it, which is what my g.p, Dr Tan and the ultrasound report recommended. On examination of my breast Dr. Sa felt the cyst and told me it was nothing. I don't need to have it removed, we will just keep check of it and he will send me for another ultrasound in three months. He said it was too small in size to do anything about it at the moment anyway. I wasn't very happy with his response. I asked questions about it and he answered them. According to Dr. Sa the cyst was simply the seroma I had after surgery and it will eventually go away.

It's very difficult to know what to say or do when you are faced with a doctor who is supposed to know what is best for you but at the same time is extremely arrogant. I didn't really understand why he never drained the seroma after surgery. Now I had a debris filled cyst and he still wanted to leave it there. My trust in Dr Sa was broken back in 2013 when I received the long lecture from him and since then he seems to get more and more arrogant. I'm sure he doesn't appreciate the fact that I ask questions. I'm supposed to take his word for it and that is it. He told me basically that I have nothing to worry about. My cancer was caught early and I'm not likely to have a recurrence. In fact, he looked out of his window, picked out a woman who was walking along the street and told me my chances of getting cancer again are no higher than hers. What a joke.

My mammogram and ultrasound results of September 2014 read – There is no abnormality in the left breast. Left breast shows no evidence of any cystic or solid lesion. Dr Sa also looked over the films of both my ultrasound and mammogram. He didn't see anything there either.

After leaving Dr. Sa's office that day I wasn't sure what to do. Should I get the second opinion like Dr. Tam suggested or do I rely on Dr. Sa and wait three months for another ultrasound? I knew which doctor's opinion I valued more and who I relied on the most but to get a second opinion meant a new specialist and most likely more tests. Although, I wanted to get that second opinion time moved quickly and I decided to wait for another ultrasound. With Christmas around the corner and other appointments to keep it was the end of January 2015 before I had another ultrasound. The ultrasound report read – There is presently an ovoid and slightly irregular hypoechoic non cystic nodule measuring 10.4mm x 3.9mm x 8.6mm lying within the dense glandular tissues beneath the surgical scar - ? Fat lobule, focal scarring or fibro adenoma. The lesion remains unchanged in size or appearance compared to the previous study.

When I compared reports it seemed to me that the latest one was incorrect. I didn't understand the meaning of some of the words used but it was clear that whatever was in my right breast had in fact grown since my last tests.

When I returned to see Dr Sa in February I was prepared for his usual attitude. I really had started to dread my appointments with Dr Sa. I felt a little sad about it as well because at the beginning he seemed like a different doctor. At this stage though there was no reason to change doctors. I hadn't even thought about it, yet. Dr Sa surprised me by reading over my ultrasound results and sending me for a biopsy. He said it was most likely nothing, but because it had changed in size it's best to have it checked. He was confident that it would be nothing to worry about. I felt relieved that Dr Sa was finally taking notice but also a little scared because he was acting on these latest results. Usually, he was quite blasé about everything, to see him change this way made me nervous, in case there really was something to worry about. If it turned out to be nothing, then I would be happy, but I wasn't confident about leaving it there and not knowing what it was.

I was so relieved after having the biopsy and returning to Dr Sa for the results to find out that the biopsy was clear. The lump in my breast, I was told, was scar tissue, not cancer, but would still be checked closely in case of any changes. I would have another ultrasound in six months' time. I was now on six monthly visits with Dr. Sa.

In May 2015, I was getting sudden, sharp pains near my lower left pelvis. The pains would come out of the blue and I would double over in pain. Dr Tam was keeping a close eye on it and also wanted me to have a pelvic ultrasound. The ultrasound results showed a cyst in the endometrium.

Every time this happens, it makes you feel as if you have just taken a few steps backwards. But, when I saw Dr Hay she told me that it's nothing to worry about. Gee, I get that a lot. It seems to be my doctors' favourite sentence. "It's nothing to worry about". The cyst was most likely caused by tamoxifen. I would have another ultrasound in three months to make sure there are no changes.

PART 2

2015. Here We Go Again – So Soon!

2015 started off well for us. We moved to a new home in a newly developed suburb. Annabelle changed to a new school. I was able to balance my appointments and treatment with less stress. Life was good for a short time.

As the year progressed we faced some hurdles. Jonathan was basically out of work, except for some casual jobs here and there. Any jobs he applied for he either didn't hear back or didn't even get to interview stage. This went on for months until he got a dream job coaching cricket at an elite school, he loved what he was doing. Hours were very limited and so was his wage. We struggled financially for a long time. I started looking for work and found a position working in child care. I only lasted 4 hours. It was too hard for me taking care of ten babies with only one other staff member. I wasn't as healthy or as fit as I thought I was and this kind of work was just too hard now. I decided to stick to my hobby of making and selling kids clothes. Finally, in April Jonathan was offered a full time position and best of all it was close to home.

Annabelle struggled at her new school. Her best friend decided not to be friends anymore and tried stopping Annabelle from making new friends. We transferred her back to her old school but she wasn't happy there either. For the first time my daughter didn't love going to school. She would cry every day and beg me not to make her go to school. For a long time she wouldn't tell me what was wrong. Then I learned that she was being bullied by a group of girls at school. They would follow her around the school, call her names and make threats. This was not only happening to Annabelle but also a few other kids at school. Annabelle by now had become close friends with another girl at school but the bullying continued. A seven year old relies on her teachers to help and support her but unfortunately in this situation the bullies were supported and protected. I had several meetings at school and was usually told what I wanted to hear but no action was ever taken against the bullies and there was never any consistency between the teachers. The bullies were able to continue their behaviours without consequences.

When it was clear to us that the school was going to ignore the situation and after going above the school to the education department with still no one acting to stop the bullying, we decided mid-year to transfer Annabelle to a new school in our local area. From day one she has been so happy there and made new friends quickly. It was the best decision we have made. She has progressed so well and has learned so much more at the new school. We have our girl back who loves school and that is such a relief.

I continued with my doctors' appointments and my

medications and zoladex implants. Our lives went on in our new "normal" mode.

Until August 2015.

On the 11th August, 2015, I had two doctors' appointments. Dr. Hay in the morning followed by an appointment with Dr. Tam. Before seeing Dr Tam, I sat in my oncologist, Dr. Hays rooms and told her that I was finally at a point in my life where I feel safe again. I feel normal. I've learned that not every new pain is cancer and I feel happy again. I don't worry anymore. That doesn't mean that I won't take notice of any changes or that I won't be vigilant. It doesn't mean that I won't take care of myself. For me it means that suddenly and very recently I let go of the fear of breast cancer returning. I'm in a good place, mentally, after two and a half years. I don't know how it happened but I was feeling happy.

Many times over the past two years I have been told by some of my medical team that my cancer was caught early and it was unlikely that it would return. I suppose a big factor also was the treatment I was on. I was continuing with tamoxifen, I had never missed a dose. I was still also having zoladex injections every four weeks.

I just thank god that my g.p Dr Tam didn't have that same attitude because once again I get to credit him with potentially saving my life. Dr Tam is always very thorough.

On the afternoon of the 11th August 2015 I saw Dr Tam because I needed a new referral for an ultrasound on my right breast to check the cyst hadn't changed. My appointment with Dr Sa was coming up in the following week and he was expecting me to bring the results but I had lost his referral. I also showed Dr Tam my pelvic ultrasound results from back in May. My pain had since stopped so I had put it out of my mind. Dr Tam said I should have a CT scan on my pelvis rather than an ultrasound because it will pick up more than an ultrasound will. Dr Tam told me that his records show that my last mammogram and ultrasound was back in February 2014. He said I was overdue for my yearly check. I told Dr Tam that I was sure I had one back in September but because he didn't have a record of it he suggested I also have a mammogram and ultrasound. It has stuck in my mind what Dr Tam said next. Dr Tam told me I should have my left breast checked because sometimes cancer can return in the other breast. He wanted my left breast checked, just to be on the safe side, just in case.

Unbelievable!

I walked out of Dr Tam's rooms with referrals for a mammogram, a bilateral breast ultrasound, a pelvic CT scan, and a pelvic ultrasound. Dr Tam's wonderful receptionist, Marley, who has become a close friend through all of this, offered to go with me for the tests. Although, I would have loved her to go with me and keep me company, I went alone because I knew she would have a long, boring wait.

Every time I have had a mammogram I have returned to the same imaging centre. This time though, I decided to go where I have my biopsies. There were a few factors for my decision. Firstly, I had to have my results for the ultrasound back fairly quickly because my appointment with Dr Sa was soon. I knew that the imaging centre where I would normally go could take weeks before I get an appointment. Secondly, I knew by having the CT scan that I would have the dye injected. I trusted the same imaging centre that I had been to previously for that. Thirdly, Marley had also been there before and suggested I go there this time too.

I phoned the imaging centre that afternoon. I had an appointment for Thursday the 13th August 2015. I certainly didn't expect to get an appointment that quick.

More Tests

I went to the imaging centre on Thursday, prepared for

a long day of tests. I wasn't particularly nervous about the results, I expected everything to come back clear. That is where I was wrong.

First up I had an internal ultrasound. If you have ever had one of those you will understand my dislike. They are uncomfortable and embarrassing. If you haven't had one, I will let you use your imagination to work out the shape and size of the handheld 'piece' that is inserted into you to obtain the best imaging.

Once I had finished having the pelvic ultrasound I waited in the waiting area to have my mammogram. This was the worse mammogram I have ever, ever had. For the first time even my left breast hurt. Both breasts getting squashed and twisted between the plates in the machine brought tears to my eyes. At the time, I blamed the woman operating the machine. She was very rough and she was quite young. I almost blurted out a few choice swear words to her. I was thinking to myself, wondering, had these women operating the mammogram machines never had a mammogram themselves? Don't they know how sensitive breasts can be? Do they not have experience or training before operating these machines? I always expect my right breast to be painful, getting squished. After all it has been through in the past two years I am getting used to the pain and discomfort but my left breast has never hurt. It's a good size and usually I don't feel anything more than a little discomfort.

When I had my breast ultrasound I was in there for much longer than I usually would be. I noticed the woman was concentrating on my left breast. I assumed that she was just being thorough. That was until she said she was finished and told me I could get dressed before she left the room. She returned a moment later and asked for my permission to do my left breast again. She said there was something that showed up in the mammogram and she wanted to make sure she found it. Of course, I laid down again and had another ultrasound. I am grateful to this woman for being upfront with me, not all people are, most of the time we are expected to wait for any results until we see our doctors. Her name was Angela, she told me that my mammogram showed a lump in my left breast. She felt the need to make sure she found it on the ultrasound too. Angela wasn't able to see it on my first ultrasound so she came back with my mammogram films and continued looking until she found the lump.

That was the moment that my world came crashing down again. A second time. My opposite breast. Just two and a half years after my first diagnosis.

Finding a lump on the scans in my left breast didn't necessarily mean that it was cancer. It could be another cyst. Thanks to Angela, though, I left the imaging centre that day aware that I was about to go through this journey for a second time. Once Angela found the lump in my breast she told me that I will need to get a biopsy as soon as possible, it didn't look good. Of course, until I had the biopsy nothing was certain.

If it wasn't for Dr. Tam always being thorough and always looking out for me and if I didn't have Angela that day of my ultrasound this new lump may not have been picked up or noticed until it was too late for me. I really wasn't due for another mammogram or ultrasound on my left side until at least February 2016. They were doing their jobs but they are both very good at it. I just wish there were more people like them.

I still had my CT scan to have, once I was done with the ultrasound. I was in shock but I also felt angry and sad. I had time to think whilst waiting for the scan and that's all I did. I knew quite well the road I was about to walk down, yet again. Not only was I in shock about what had just taken place but I was still nervous about having the c.t scan, particularly about the dye that will be injected. I had a short wait before having the cannula inserted into my arm. My left arm has been used so much over the last couple of years for blood tests and such that my veins aren't as good as they once were, it can take a few attempts to get a good vein and, of course, that is what happened.

Finally, I was taken into the room for the c.t scan. I waited for the dye to be inserted into the cannula followed by the rush of heat. Thankfully, it was over in no time and I was able to have the cannula removed and get dressed. I had been there, at the imaging centre, for five hours. Now, I was on my way to pick up my girl from school.

The Unexpected but Always Feared

For the past two and a half years I have lived in fear of cancer returning. Until recently every new ache or pain scared me. I often lay awake thinking about cancer returning and my chances of survival, if it did. I was told early on that my first cancer was fast growing and the only way is up, so if it was to return, chances are it would be too late for me unless it was caught early. In my mind, having a double mastectomy was something I have recently started thinking about but cancer can still get in the remaining tissue or bones and it can pop up anywhere else anyway. It has always been on my mind that the cancer will return but I relied on my treatment to keep me safe, to keep the cancer away. I always thought, when it returned it would be in my bones, same breast or elsewhere. I never thought much about getting it in the other breast. I never thought I would have a recurrence so soon.

I picked up my results from the imaging centre the next day. I had made an appointment to see Dr. Tam but I also decided to have a read myself before I saw him. My results were surprising, to say the least.

Mammogram – Within the inner superior quadrant of the breast, a small nodule is demonstrated, which measure up to 7mm.

Bilateral Breast Ultrasound – In the right breast at 10 o'clock position 20mm from the nipple, the 14 x 5 x 8mm well-defined hypoechic structure shows no significant change in size compared to ultrasound of February 2015.

The left breast at the 10 o'clock position 90mm from the nipple, shows a 7 x 5 x 5mm hypoechic structure with posterior shadowing and an echogenic halo is demonstrated. This is suspicious for a breast mitotic lesion. Ultrasound guided biopsy is recommended.

Pelvic Ultrasound – The endometrium shows a thickness of up to 6mm and shows three cysts. This is likely related to tamoxifen therapy.

CT Abdomen – clear.

As you do, but never should, I took to google to find out what it all meant. Everything pointed towards breast cancer in my left breast.

I saw Dr Tam that afternoon. We discussed my results. Dr Tam apologised and said it doesn't look good. He was genuinely upset by the report and the fact that he thought I now had breast cancer in my left breast. He was also concerned about the cysts I had. Knowing that I was seeing Dr Sa next week, he had one piece of advice for me, if Dr Sa does not act immediately on this then he is willing to refer me to someone else. He told me to remember how important it is to act quickly. Dr Tam was well aware of how Dr Sa has acted and responded in the past, so he wanted me to be confident when seeing him that I was able to change if I felt I wanted to. Dr Tam actually offered to give me a new referral for another doctor then and there but I decided to see Dr Sa again. Sometimes it feels better to stick to who you know. I would see Dr Tam again after I see Dr Sa.

Goodbye to the arrogant

I remember, back in 2013, when I was booking my first surgery with Dr Sa's receptionist, Lola, she told me, "Dr. Sa is going to be THE BEST breast Surgeon in Australia within five years". Lola said, "Don't worry you are in great hands, ladies don't even have any pain afterwards and you won't even see your scar". Well, I admit my scar is good and yes I do believe he is a good surgeon but I think Dr. Sa has the same beliefs as his receptionist and has let his inspirations of being 'the best' get in the way. I believe Dr. Sa unfortunately, has forgotten how to treat a patient. He has lost his charm, his bedside manner and has forgotten how to communicate with people in a positive manner. It's a shame when someone changes for the worse and can put money and a drive to be 'the best' ahead of anything else. I feel for his patients who will continue to see him. The people who want to but don't have the strength, courage or mindset to change doctors.

A week after having my scans, on August 20th, I had my appointment with Dr. Sa. I didn't go to my appointment planning on changing doctors. I was a little nervous, as I have been for every appointment with him since the lecture he gave me about having chemo. I was concerned that he may not act, that he might respond with his usual 'it's nothing', but I had no idea what I was in for. For my previous appointment with Dr. Sa, Jonathan and Annabelle were with me but this time I was alone, giving Dr. Sa a better opportunity to treat me the way he did.

Dr. Sa welcomed me with his usual, 'how are you', this time my response was, well, not the best and I handed him my reports from my scans. Dr. Sa now uses a recorder and speaks into it throughout the visit. He reported my cancer history into the recorder whilst he browsed my reports. He always mentions the fact that I had only one cycle of chemotherapy due to the fact that I was unable to tolerate it. That comment always makes me smirk. After pausing the recorder he put my films up, under the light and browsed them. At first, I thought I was speaking with the old doctor but that quickly changed.

Dr. Sa spoke to me whilst looking over my films. He told me that it was possible this was cancer again. I know the drill, I will have to have a biopsy to find out for sure. He said the good news is that we have caught it early because the lump is a small size. Worst case scenario, I will have surgery again, best case it will turn out to be a cyst or similar.

Dr Sa then asked me to undress so he could check my breasts, something he does on every visit.
He said, "It's nothing. I can't feel anything, so it's no big

deal. " He told me to get dressed as he returned to his desk. As I was putting my top back on Dr. Sa then said something that I will never forget. He said, "I suppose you are feeling sorry for yourself and asking yourself, why me? This is nothing, do you know those old men that go and have their skin cancers removed? The surgery is nothing more than a scrape on the arm and it's gone. That's exactly what this is, it's nothing". Then he sat at his desk and waited for me to take my seat.

I couldn't believe what I just heard, from a breast cancer surgeon. On one hand he is telling me I most likely have cancer again and then he is telling me it's nothing. How can cancer, in any form, be nothing? There are so many reasons to be concerned, for him to also be concerned, about a return of cancer in such a short period of time. Instead of attacking me, he should be explaining to me how this could happen. I just don't understand his attitude.

My response was, "I think if this is breast cancer then I have every right to feel sorry for myself and ask why me! I am not feeling that way right now, I'm actually feeling quite angry, but why shouldn't I? This is my second time in two and a half years. I haven't even recovered from the first time yet. For the past two years I have been told that it was unlikely to come back but yet here I am again. You might think breast cancer is nothing worse than a scrape on the arm but I remember very well what I went through and exactly how it felt".

Dr. Sa then continued on, he told me he has many women coming into see him who have no chance left in life. They have no choice but to lose their breasts. The remainder of their lives are very limited, their cancers were not caught early, like mine. He said I should feel lucky. These other women would give anything to be in my situation.

Those comments made my blood boil and I wish now, looking back that I had walked out on him right then.

Instead, I told him that I know too well exactly how it is to be told you have no chance. I reminded him that I have lost my mum and sister to cancer. I said I know that I am not in the same category as those other women but that doesn't mean I don't have the right to be worried or to think "why me". I never want to be in the same situation as the other women and you obviously don't know if cancer will keep returning over and over again.

I strongly believe, although I tested inconclusive to the BRCA genes that there must be something else that is causing cancer in my family. I asked Dr. Sa if I could become a guinea pig for genetic testing and help in some way to possibly find other genetic links to breast cancer or to have tests done for other mutations. Dr. Sa had told me previously about his close links with the hospital that specialises in genetic testing. I have heard of other genes that have been linked to breast cancer, but every time I question that, I am told there are no other genetic links that Australia is aware of. I have only been tested for the BRCA1 and BRCA2 gene mutations, but I am aware of many women who have been tested for other mutations. Unfortunately, I was met with more of the same attitude from Dr. Sa. He told me we have thousands of genes in our bodies and it would be impossible to test me. He actually laughed at me but I pushed it a little further by mentioning the gene mutations that I am aware of. But again he basically repeated himself and made it clear that my time with him was up, by standing and heading for the door.

Dr. Sa was at least sending me for a biopsy which his receptionist booked me in for. My appointment was made for that same afternoon. I was expected to return to see Dr. Sa the following week.

Biopsy

I had to go directly back to the imaging centre where I had recently had my scans to have a biopsy. I was so upset about Dr Sa's attitude but I had to put it to the back of my mind so I could prepare myself for the biopsy and get there safely.

When I arrived for my appointment I was relieved to see a new sign. The sign read that results of any tests can also be emailed directly to a doctor of your choice if the centre is advised on booking in. I asked the lady on the desk to please forward my results to Dr. Tam. I had a week to wait before seeing Dr. Sa again and I knew there was a good chance that Dr. Tam would have them sooner. Waiting a week for biopsy results is so stressful. The not knowing is one of the hardest steps in the breast cancer process.

This time my biopsy was a little different. I had a core biopsy and also an ultrasound guided fine needle aspiration biopsy. The process was much longer this time and a lot more uncomfortable. I was given extra doses of the anaesthetic because each time the doctor tested my breast for numbness I still had feeling. The fine-needle aspiration is guided by ultrasound, when the needle is inserted into the breast and in to the lump to remove some fluid for testing. I had two needles of fluid removed. Next, I had the core biopsy, when tissue is removed through the hollow needle. When the tissue has been collected there is a large bang. The bang sound of the needle still unsettles me. I try not to look but it was difficult this time and being my third or fourth biopsy I am slowly getting used to them.

Always My Shoulder to Cry On.

  Throughout my whole journey I have had just one person always by my side and always ready to listen to me no matter what. He is my shoulder to cry on when things get too tough, we laugh together and cry together. I know I can rely on him. We argue, just like any couple, our relationship isn't perfect but we are definitely closer now. Without him by my side I know this journey would have been more difficult and I really don't know how I would have come through it without my husband, Jonathan. He hears all me fears and worries and I hear his, quite often the partner or loved one is forgotten during cancer, but I often see the worry in him. I am blessed to have both Jonathan and Annabelle, without them I would have nothing.

  After having the biopsy, that evening, Jonathan and I had a long talk and made some decisions. We wouldn't tell Annabelle until we knew exactly what was happening and she would have as little information as possible. During the bullying incidents at her old school, we had to take her to see a psychologist because of the anxiety it was causing. Our girl had just recently returned to her beautiful self, so we wanted to upset her as little as possible.

We both knew that I couldn't and shouldn't return to see Dr. Sa, we both agreed that I would see a new surgeon, regardless of the outcome of the biopsy. Jonathan had been to many of my appointments with Dr. Sa, so he was well aware of his attitude and arrogance. The last appointment I had was the last straw for me, emotionally I could not walk into his rooms again. I could not allow that doctor to operate on me. Dealing with a diagnosis of cancer was hard enough, but having to deal also with people like him was too much. It was a relief to have Jonathans support on this, because the thought of seeing Dr. Sa again was making me feel ill. He over stepped this time. I feel that what he said to me that day, should never be said to a patient by any doctor. We agreed to wait for Dr. Tam to call me in for the biopsy results and have him refer me to someone else. Jonathan would make the call to Dr. Sa to tell them I won't be returning.

We discussed how we felt about this. We knew there was only a tiny chance of it not being cancer. At the time, I thought it would be easier for me this time because I knew what to expect.

Jonathan kept his Mum and Dad up to date, every step of the way. As always, they were there for us. They offered to do what they can, they have always been a great support to us. I'm glad Jonathan has them to lean on, sometimes he has needed that extra person in his life just to talk to.

Jonathan made the call to Dr. Sa's rooms the day after we received my biopsy results. He spoke with Lola and told her I wouldn't be returning to Dr. Sa. Lola was a little shocked and wanted to know the reason, so Jonathan told her it was basically because of the way I was spoken to by Dr. Sa and his attitude towards me. Jonathan told Lola a little of what Dr. Sa had said to me. Lola's response was that she had never received any complaint about Dr. Sa before, not ever and I don't think she really believed it. She was being loyal to her boss. She wished us all the best and told Jonathan to make sure I have a new doctor as soon as possible and to follow up on my results from the biopsy, it's very important and quite urgent. Obviously, by Lola's comments, they also already had my biopsy results and she was making sure that we knew how important it was to seek a new doctor. I don't hold any ill feelings against Lola, she is a lovely lady.

Biopsy Results

As soon as Dr. Tam received my biopsy results, on 24th August, he called me in to see him, to go through them with me. I am so relieved now that I had the results sent to Dr. Tam.

Dr Tam read through the results and then told me I had cancer in my left breast. Seeing the look on his face just made me feel sad. He was upset for me, again. We discussed the results which were-

The breast core biopsies shows the presence of an **infiltrating ductal carcinoma. Malignant** luminal calcifications are identified associated with the **tumour.**

Ancillary Tests:
ER: Positive (3+ in 99%)
PR: Positive (2-3+ in 60%)
HER2 – IHC: Equivocal (1-2+ staining)
P63: Negative, confirming the invasive nature
Ki67 index: 7%

Summary

Left breast, 10 o' clock, 9cm fn:

- **invasive ductal carcinoma nst; ER and PR positive**

The most shocking part of that report for me wasn't that I had cancer in my left breast. When I saw er+ and pr+ I couldn't believe my eyes. Dr. Tam explained the results but I already understood. We discussed the fact that the cancer is again er+ and pr+, I think we were both in shock. I was feeling a little angry about that. Dr. Tam, being a general practitioner, doesn't have the expertise of an oncologist, but in saying that I find him to be very knowledgeable in all areas and I put all my trust in him. We discussed my recent appointment with Dr. Sa and I told Dr. Tam what was said to me. Immediately, Dr. Tam told me he will refer me to a new surgeon. He agreed that I should never have been spoken to in that way, especially by a doctor. Dr. Tam was angry with me about the treatment I received from Dr. Sa. I suspect he will no longer be referring any patients to Dr. Sa in the future.

As Dr Tam printed my referral for my new surgeon he also told me if I wasn't happy with this doctor he can easily refer me elsewhere. He wanted to ensure that I felt comfortable with the doctor and it didn't matter if it took several referrals and doctors.

Family and Friends

  Telling family and friends is one of the hardest things to do. This time I put it off for as long as possible. I was reluctant to tell anybody and seriously considered telling only those people very close to us. It wasn't that it was a secret, I just find it difficult to say those words and never knowing how people will react is also difficult. Being my second time with cancer within two and a half years I think I expected most people to react differently compared to the first time. I have never looked for sympathy from anyone but a little consideration goes a long way.

  Having cancer can change relationships with the people in your life. I've read and heard other people speak of the distance a cancer diagnosis brings. When treatment ends, family and friends are often not prepared for the fact that recovery takes time. In general, your recovery will take much longer than your treatment did. Many people assume once surgery and initial treatment is over, you are cured and life goes back to normal. Life only goes back to normal for those who are not directly affected by the cancer diagnosis.

  For two and a half years I have struggled with medications, side effects, aches and pains caused by those medications and most of all menopause. Rarely does a week go by that I don't have a doctor's appointment. I have had so many scans and blood tests in two and a half years that I have lost count. I always had good veins pre-cancer, now they are difficult to find. I've even had blood taken from veins in my feet. I've gained 50 kilograms since chemo. I've lived everyday wondering when will the cancer come back and where will it pop up this time. Now, I also live with breasts that are of significant difference in size. There is no hiding that. On one side I am almost flat chested, nothing more than a small handful. The other side is huge, probably an E cup. It hurts to wear a bra. So, I leave the house when I have to because I never actually want to. I would be happy not leaving the house or going out in public at all. If I can avoid going anywhere, I will. The only place I am comfortable going is to our local club for the meat raffle and that is only because I can sit in an almost empty room. The club is small and not busy at all.

There were some friends and family who I didn't want to tell. I was tempted to make a post on facebook but I thought that would be heartless, I felt a responsibility to tell people, so reluctantly I told them that my cancer had returned. Some people I was able to tell face to face, other people I had to tell by phone. Some people's reactions just made me regret telling them at all.

If you can't find it within yourself to show that you care, even a little. If you think it is an opportunity for you to make the conversation about yourself, your fears, and your health or if you have nothing to say whatsoever then that is a reflection on you. That shows your selfishness and it only pushes away the people who always cared about you. It's never a competition, you can't compete with a cancer diagnosis, worrying that you might get it or thinking you have it, does not compare to actually having cancer. Being diagnosed with cancer is frightening to say the least.

The one thing cancer teaches you is that life is too short to worry about those who are selfish and self-involved. Cancer teaches you to keep close those that you love and those that love you. It is quite common, unfortunately, that a cancer diagnosis tears friendships and families apart.

One of the excuses often used is that people don't know what to say or do. What's so hard to simply send a text message asking, how are you? Why can't you ask what happened at the doctor's appointment? During a conversation why can't you just ask a question? People who don't make any effort at all simply show that they don't care.

It's not possible to know why certain people are unable to offer even minimal support. Some people react to bad news as if it were contagious. When you are frightened, when you are struggling, when you most need their support, they disappear. If this happens to you, if people vanish, although we all would like to know why these people made themselves scarce, you eventually learn that it doesn't really matter. It is more important for us to focus on our health.

I read on a personal blog recently that it is quite common for people to assume that family and friends gather around after a diagnosis. Homes are full of flowers and cards. Meals are cooked for the family. When you are not able to drive there is always someone there volunteering to get you to that appointment. It didn't happen at all for that blogger nor for many people in some of the groups I belong to. Some people are quite young, only in their twenties or have small children. Their partners are of not much help or leave. Their close family and friends vanish. I often hear that once surgery and chemo are finished so are the offers of assistance.

Many people agree they sometimes feel they are not listened to or are not allowed to speak about how they are feeling or what they are going through. Unfortunately, this is common and I often feel that way myself.

I think it is more common to fight this alone than it is to be surrounded by people. That is where the smaller charities are of great assistance. Some will offer cleaners to come in and clean the home, or grocery vouchers. Some will even help out with bills, because anyone who has cancer will know exactly how expensive it can be.

I have always been blessed that I have Jonathan by my side but I really feel for those people who are alone. If you have at least one strong person by your side then you don't need the other people who walked away or choose to ignore you.

Starting Over

I started searching for as much information as I could get about my new breast surgeon. I wanted the best, but I also wanted a doctor who doesn't have the ego and arrogance of Dr. Sa. I was very nervous and anxious about meeting a new doctor. I posted in one of the Facebook groups that I belong to, asking if anyone was a patient of my new surgeon. A couple of ladies were, they had good things to say about him which helped me to relax a little.

From my google searching, I learned that my new doctor had many years of experience. He operates in several hospitals including the private hospital close to my home. He holds a high position at one of Sydney's biggest public hospitals and has devoted his professional life to cancer.

I had my first appointment with my new surgeon, Dr. Campbell, on the 31st August, 2015. To say I was nervous was an understatement. So many things were going through my head as I waited for Dr. Campbell. I was concerned that he might know Dr. Sa and might be unhappy that I changed doctors. All I wished for was a doctor to be professional, to be good at his job and to give me his opinion as a doctor. I didn't need nice or friendly, not even caring really, although that would be a bonus.

I learned a few things by seeing Dr. Campbell. The first one being that I should have changed to him a long time ago. I wish he had been my surgeon from the start. Dr. Campbell is very experienced and really knows what he is talking about. He is quite pleasant without being over the top. He is not money hungry at all, that became quite obvious to me almost straight away. He takes care to see what others might have missed. He doesn't appreciate other doctors who over charge their patients, especially when they don't deliver what they promise or charge for.

Dr. Campbell read through my referral and my reports, he asked me questions about my history. He looked at my most recent mammogram and ultrasound results, he then also looked at my previous results. Comparing them under the light Dr Campbell then said something that shook me.

Dr. Campbell showed me both my most recent mammogram and the one previously. The lump in my left breast also showed up in my previous mammogram. The cancer in my left breast had been there for at least six months, but no doctor, nobody, had seen it. It had slipped by un-noticed. When Dr. Campbell pointed it out to me I could see it clearly. My heart stopped. Knowing that it had been there for so long could mean that this is much more serious than I expected. Now the fear was setting in.

Dr. Campbell asked about the cancer in my right

breast. He wanted to know what surgery I had done and by whom. I was nervous about discussing Dr. Sa but I was surprised and relieved about Dr. Campbell's response.

I told Dr. Campbell that I had a 'partial mastectomy' on my right breast.

He asked, "What's that?".

I thought, that was a very odd question. I was confused by it because I had seen and heard the words used many times. I hesitated with my answer and was wondering, how could he not know what a partial mastectomy is?

I told him I had the cancer and tissue around it removed.

Dr. Campbell said, "Well, we all do that!".

I said I also had a lift and mammoplasty (to increase the size of my breast).

Dr. Campbell said, "And let me guess, he charged you a fortune for it."

I told Dr. Campbell that yes, I had paid about $5500 and had my surgery in a public hospital. Dr. Campbell appeared very annoyed about that. I also picked up that Dr. Campbell had heard the name of Dr. Sa before and wasn't impressed by that surgeon. I felt there was not only annoyance but possibly anger too. I suspect they either have a history or Dr. Sa is not looked upon in a high regard among his colleagues. I was feeling more and more confident that I had made the right decision by leaving Dr. Sa and certain that I am not the first patient of his to do it, neither will I be the last.

Dr. Campbell then did a breast examination, he was able to feel the lump in my left breast. He also examined my right breast. Dr. Campbell had me repeat to him what exactly I thought Dr Sa did when he operated on me. I again told him that I had a partial mastectomy including a mammoplasty. Dr. Campbell then told me something I never expected to hear, ever!

Dr. Campbell told me that there is nothing in my right breast. There is no implant. I received a lumpectomy and that is all. I was so shocked. I still am. I really just can't find the words. If Dr. Campbell is right?

My thoughts on this are:

Although I was originally told there is a big difference between a partial mastectomy and a lumpectomy, I think they are the same thing. Partial mastectomy is just the new, more fashionable word used for lumpectomy, more so by the younger doctors coming through, the term lumpectomy still being used by the senior doctors. It all gets quite confusing but when you add to that mammoplasty then things change a little because mammoplasty means-plastic surgery of the breast; **augmentation mamm oplasty** plastic surgery to increase the size of the f emale breast, or sometimes to uplift pendulous breasts.

To enlarge a breast, a saline filled or silicone gel prosthesis is inserted in a pocke t formed beneath the breast on the chest wall.

I was billed for and told I was having a partial mastectomy plus mammoplasty. To now be told by a different doctor that I did not receive that confirms I definitely made the right decision changing doctors. Whether I can do or say anything about that legally is something I will consider finding out later down the track.

We returned to Dr. Campbell's desk to discuss the next step. Dr. Campbell answered my questions and gave me exactly enough information. I was prepared to have a mastectomy or double mastectomy this time. I really don't want to have to go through this again. Dr. Campbell told me he would do that for me if I'm certain it's what I want. He told me that he didn't think I had to do it, removing the lump and tissue around it, in his opinion would be enough. Dr. Campbell was hoping the cancer was slow growing and we had caught it early enough for it not to have spread elsewhere. He told me that although I had been on estrogen blockers for 2 years, it is very unusual, and only happens in 4% of people that the same type of cancer returns.

I again decided to have the lumpectomy. I don't know if it is the right decision. Perhaps I will be unlucky and get it a 3rd time but that can happen with or without breasts. Removing my breasts doesn't stop the cancer from coming back again. It can still get in the chest wall and any muscle or tissue that remains. It can also metastasis to elsewhere in my body. To be honest I think I was too scared to have a mastectomy. A lumpectomy/partial mastectomy is what I know. I know what to expect and at the time that is how I coped with my second diagnosis. By thinking that I knew what to expect because I had already been through it before, that is how I coped.

Dr. Campbell checked his diary and booked me in for surgery for his first available day. He told me since I was in private health that I could have my surgery in the private hospital. He told me I wouldn't have any expenses for the surgery because he doesn't charge above the threshold. I wouldn't have to do or pay anything. He will handle all claims. The only thing I have to do is prepare myself for surgery. The next best thing I heard was that Dr. Campbell will operate in the morning so I could go home by that evening, if all goes well. I was so happy about that because I really don't like hospitals and having to be away from my family. I wanted this over as quickly as possible so I could heal and start over again.

However, Dr. Campbell did also say that this surgery may not be as simple or straight forward as my last. Dr. Campbell explained that if the lymph nodes involved are under my arm then they will be removed during surgery but because my lump is in my left breast and is close to my chest wall it is possible that the sentinel lymph node will be located in the middle of my chest, on my chest wall. My surgery then becomes more complicated and the lymph node/s on my chest wall will be removed. If this occurs my stay in hospital could be for several nights.

Dr. Campbell made an appointment for me to have a c.t scan and sentinel node mapping done on 15th September 2015. He explained it could take up to 5 hours as it is a long process. I would have that done at a hospital in Sydney then come back afterwards to the private hospital and have the hook wire inserted, ready for my surgery to take place on the 16th September 2015. I also had to stop taking tamoxifen immediately because that can cause blood clots.

Lymphoscintigraphy (sentinel lymph node mapping) is an imaging technique used to identify the lymph drainage basin, determine the number of sentinel nodes, differentiate sentinel nodes from subsequent nodes, locate the sentinel node in an unexpected location, and mark the sentinel node over the skin for biopsy.

Sentinel node mapping is rapidly becoming an alternate staging procedure for the axilla in managing early breast cancer. Several well-conducted studies have provided high-quality evidence for its usefulness. Sentinel node scanning was initially studied in cutaneous melanomas to detect lymphatic drainage patterns prior to surgery. The procedure is applicable to almost all regions of the body, but the greatest impetus to the technique came with the application of the procedure to identify breast sentinel nodes.

The sentinel node is the first node to receive metastatic deposits in a malignancy. Lymphoscintigraphy is an important procedure because if the sentinel node is free of metastasis, subsequent nodes are also likely to be free of disease. The sentinel node is generally defined as follows:

- The node closest to the primary lesion
- The node with a radioactive channel leading to it
- The node with the highest count rate on lymphoscintigraphic imaging and probe counting
- The first node visible on lymphoscintigraphic imaging
- The blue node on dye injection technique
- The node with a blue channel leading to it
  Source - http://emedicine.medscape.com

Surgery

My surgery was booked for late in the morning on the 16th of September but I received a call a few days before from Dr. Campbell's receptionist to change the time of surgery. Dr. Campbell wanted to operate early in the morning, about 7am, therefore I had to stay overnight in hospital, before the surgery, because it was too early in the morning to go in on the day. I would still be having the preparations for surgery done on the 15th, so it was going to be a very busy day.

I would be alone this time. Jonathan had taken a couple of days off work but he would have to get Annabelle to school and take care of her.

A couple of days before surgery I was barely able to move. I had such severe pain in my shoulder and across my neck and upper back. We called an ambulance the night before my surgery because I was unable to move. My neck, shoulder and back had locked and I was in excruciating pain. I chose not to go to hospital because the ambos' were able to explain to us what was happening and if I went to hospital my surgery would be cancelled. Apparently, the pain was related to the breast cancer and it happens often to people both before and after surgery. I would need strong pain relief and steroids. This is yet another unwanted side effect of cancer.

On the morning of the 15th September 2015, Jonathan, Annabelle and I left for the hospital medical centre in the city. My bag was packed and I was as prepared as I could be for the long day ahead.

I had to have the mapping done first which consisted of scans and injections and a blood test. After each test was completed I would have to return to the waiting room and wait to be called for the next one. Jonathan and Annabelle stayed in the waiting room and only left to buy themselves some lunch or a drink. I was still struggling to move freely so I would have to ask to be helped up after each scan. Once I was done I had to wait to collect the results, which took over an hour. By the time I was finished it was close to 5pm and I was running late to have the hook wire done at the private hospital.

We were all tired after a terribly long day. I was feeling guilty that Annabelle and Jonathan had been sitting in the waiting room most of the day. When we returned to the car and had to pay the parking fee of $78 we couldn't believe it. The car park is located at a public hospital and we had been parked there for under 5 hours. The rates are shocking and I can't remember now if we even noticed on entry the sign listing the fees for parking. We were just lucky that we actually had enough money with us at the time.

As we headed to the private hospital, about an hour drive in peak hour traffic, staff from the hospital phoned to check that I was still coming. I was late now for my appointment to have the hook wire inserted and to be admitted to the ward. We were still at least 30 minutes away but I was told they will wait for me.

When we arrived at the hospital, staff were waiting for us at reception and took me straight through for the tests. I thought I was prepared and ready for the hook wire because I had it done for my last surgery. This time it was done a little differently. First I had a mammogram of my left breast. Not being able to move my upper body without pain and having my breast squished in the machine hurt like hell. The lady wasn't impressed that she was still at work and should have finished earlier. So she just shoved my body into place, in a hurry, not being gentle at all and not taking any time with it. She wanted out of there and I was to blame for her still being at work. She used the old machine but once she had me in place and went to take pictures she realized the machine wasn't working. We had to do it all over again in another room on another machine. This time I told her to take it easy. I was past caring by then whether I was being rude or not she was hurting me but she couldn't care less.

After the mammogram I was then led to another room for an ultrasound and the hook wire. I remember the first time I had it done how much difficulty they had doing it. I also remember having an anesthetic inserted first. Not this time, this time my breast was wiped with a type of anesthetic and guided by the ultrasound, the wire was inserted with a large needle through my breast and into the lump. The wire had to be wriggled around until it hooked onto the lump in my breast. I closed my eyes, held my breath and waited for it to be over.

I then had to go to admissions to sign into hospital and go to the ward. I felt like I had been beaten up a bit today. I was exhausted and in pain. I was grateful once I got to my room that it was a single room. I just wanted to rest and not be bothered by anybody else. I handed over my medications to the nurse on my ward. The pain medication I kept. I didn't trust them to give me medication for pain when I needed it. I had to be nil by mouth by midnight. The nurse gave me surgical stockings to put on and leave on. When my blood pressure was checked, it was very low. That is very unusual because since my first diagnosis I have been on medication for high blood pressure. I hadn't yet had my medication for blood pressure. The doctor was called to come in and discuss what to do.

Jonathan and Annabelle had such a long day, as much as I wanted them to stay as long as possible, after a short time I sent them home. They were tired too and needed to eat and relax. I wouldn't see them again until after surgery the next day when I am returned to my room. I didn't want either of them to see me cry so I held back my tears until they were gone.

I was feeling very nervous and tired. When the doctor

arrived and again checked my blood pressure, it was still very low. The doctor told me not to have my medication and if it doesn't go up I will not be able to have surgery.

I slept that night in patches, waking up every hour or so and watching the clock. I wanted this over but at the same time I was getting very anxious. I was alone and I was scared. Every thought went through my head. What if I don't wake up after surgery? What if the cancer has spread? Mostly, I prayed that the lymph nodes would be removed from only under my arm so I could go home after surgery.

By 6am I was up and prepared for surgery. Shortly after, I was taken down to the operating rooms by the nurses and wards man. I faintly remember their conversation about an overseas holiday. I had entered the place in my head where I was a little spaced out. Knowing what was happening but not really being there. I tried to think of other things and not my surgery.

My blood pressure was checked several more times, it was still low but had risen to an appropriate number. I was placed in the waiting bay, outside the operating room, for what seemed like an eternity. A cannula was inserted in my arm ready for the anesthetic .To remind all theatre staff that I was unable to have any bloods or blood pressure taken from my right arm, due to my previous surgery and removal of lymph nodes, an arm band was placed on my arm. If my right arm is used it could cause lymphedema.

I was taken into the operating theatre, moved onto the bed. I remember the anesthetist telling me he was inserting the anesthetic and then I woke up in recovery. It was over. Once again the cancer had been removed.

Once I was awake and my vitals were normal I was moved back to my room. Jonathan and Annabelle were there waiting for me. They had been waiting for a couple of hours. I was so happy to see them. I couldn't control my tears and cried a little.

I don't remember feeling any pain. All I remember is once I was awake properly I wanted to go home. I had to wait for the doctor to see me and if all went well then I could leave. It was a few hours before I was able to get up and out of the bed. I was very groggy and very thirsty.

Dr. Campbell came in to see me later in the afternoon. I don't remember much of the conversation, only that all the cancer was removed and I had two lymph nodes removed. One from my chest wall and the other from under my arm, both were clear of cancer. Thank goodness. Dr. Campbell told me since I look so well and he can see that I am eager to go home I can go as soon as my paper work is completed. I see him again in two weeks.

Recovery

Dealing with having cancer for the second time wasn't as easy as I first thought. It was different for me because I knew what the process was but it wasn't as easy as I thought it would be. In fact, it has been much harder this time.

The worry about cancer returning has doubled, now I really do live in fear that if or when it returns I won't be as lucky as what I have been.

On my return visit to Dr. Campbell after surgery he gave me some great news. It was a grade 1 cancer, meaning it was small and slow growing. Although I had prepared myself for chemo I wouldn't be having it. I would only need to have radiation this time. My next visit with Dr. Campbell would be in six months, because I was healing and coping very well.

However, a week after that appointment with Dr. Campbell I developed an infection and swelling under my left arm. Dr. Tam tried treating it with antibiotics but it was getting worse rather than better. I had to attend emergency at the hospital where Dr. Campbell practices, unfortunately, he was on holidays at the time. There was some confusion at the hospital as to who should be seeing me. I had a letter from Dr. Tam to give to emergency explaining that he had already been in contact with Dr. Campbell and I was to see his registrar on arrival. Somehow that didn't get passed on, so after waiting 4 hours and still not being seen by anyone we left at midnight.

The next day I went to the emergency at our local hospital. I was in pain, not able to move my arm and the swelling and redness was getting worse. I assumed, wrongly, that a needle would be put in to drain the fluid. I was taken for an ultrasound and seen by a general surgeon in emergency. I was told I had to be admitted and have emergency surgery that evening. The wound would be opened with a drain put in place and it would remain open for several days. Apparently, that was the only way to clear the fluid and infection. I agreed to have the surgery, signed papers and after several hours in emergency I was moved to a ward.

That was when I fell apart. It all became too much for me as soon as I entered the room. I sat on the bed and cried. I told Jonathan that I couldn't do it. I couldn't have the surgery and I couldn't stay in the hospital. I wasn't able to stay in that room with the other patients, there were three other people, it was a four bed room. I started to panic, thinking I would have to have the surgery. As soon as a nurse came in to see me I told her I couldn't stay, I had changed my mind, but she didn't understand English very well and had no idea what I was saying. I asked her to send in another nurse. As other nurses came in I continued crying and panicking. I was told I had to stay. I was told I had signed the papers for surgery already and they will be coming to get me very soon. They sent doctors in to see me. I argued with one doctor because he wanted to know why I had changed my mind. I was honest with him about how I was feeling. I told him I was scared that it was the wrong thing to do. I told him that I just don't have the strength, I've had enough, I just can't do anymore. I told him I want to go home. I also told him that my mum had been in this ward and I just can't stay here. He didn't seem to understand, he was very rude and told me that I could go home and die without having the surgery. He told me I was being stupid. The more I stood my ground, the angrier he became so I refused to change my mind and became angry with him. He told me until the surgeons are finished and come to see me I can't leave. Other nurses also came in to change my mind, trying to tell me that I will die without this surgery. Telling me the doctors have stayed back in theatre especially to operate on me. I knew that was a lie. I was still waiting for surgery because they were still operating on other emergencies. When they couldn't change my mind about going home they sent the surgeon in to see me. I had to explain how I was feeling all over again and why I was feeling the way I was. She told me having this surgery is the only way to remove the fluid and heal the infection. She tried hard to change my mind even offering me a room to myself. At one point I had five medical staff at my bed trying to force me into having the surgery, they even tried telling me it was too late to back out or change my mind because I had already signed the papers for the surgery. At that point, I demanded that my cannula be removed or I would remove it myself. I told them that they cannot force me to stay in hospital or have surgery. I told them I am going home. Two hours later, my cannula was removed and I went home.

I just knew, I had a terribly bad feeling that they were wrong. I was overcome with emotion. I couldn't control how I was feeling. I just knew I couldn't, shouldn't have that surgery and I had to go home. There is no way possible I could have had that surgery. I had the worse feeling in my stomach and I knew I had to get out of there. Not one of the nurses or doctors understood my decision. They could see how distressed I was yet they still pushed and insisted. Maybe they have never seen anybody so upset and scared before. I don't understand why they were all insisting on the surgery and why they were so rude and angry with me. I only hope that it had nothing at all to do with my private health insurance funds being paid to the hospital for the surgery and my stay in the hospital.

A week later I was contacted by the hospital asking me to give approval for the hospital to claim through my private health fund for my stay and treatment in the hospital. He explained how important it was to the hospital to receive these extra funds, when possible.

They wanted to claim $3000 from my health fund. I told him to double check his information because I didn't stay in hospital nor did I have treatment. Then when he has the correct information he can send me the papers to sign. I never received the papers.

As it turned out I was right about the surgery. The next day I returned to Dr. Tam. He understood immediately why I was feeling that way. He said I had no trust in the surgeons because I didn't know them and it is not their area of expertise. He again contacted Dr. Campbell, whilst he was still on holidays, explained the situation and again Dr. Campbell told me to return to his hospital to see his registrar.

On the Monday morning Jonathan and I returned to Dr. Campbell's practicing hospital in the city. I explained that I was there on Friday night but returned home before being seen. I told them that the registrar of Dr. Campbell was waiting to see me. Finally, after a short wait I was seen by Dr. Thoung the registrar of Dr. Campbell. He checked my breast and underarm, had bloods taken and contacted Dr. Campbell. I was sent to have an ultrasound. The decision was made to have it drained by ultrasound guided needle. A syringe would be inserted into the area and they would drain as much fluid as possible. We waited a few hours in emergency for a doctor to be available.

I was taken to a small room in the emergency

department. The doctor explained what would happen today. I would be given a local anesthetic, inserted into my underarm. Using the ultrasound to guide them, a small cut would be made and he would then insert the needle and withdraw as much fluid as possible. There was no pain, it was a little uncomfortable. I could feel the fluid being drained and the doctor enjoyed telling me what was happening. He knew I couldn't look because I was squeamish but he thought I should know the details. Thanks doctor. Gross. They were able to extract 90ml today, most of the fluid under my arm. The process took about half an hour. Dr.Thoung came in the room before we were finished. Both doctors were very pleasant. Their sense of humour made the process that little bit easier.

Once I was finished my arm was padded and taped up. I was given antibiotics and pain relief. I was given an appointment in two days' time at the cancer centre at the same hospital to see Dr. Thoung. Finally, after another long day we were able to go home. I was already feeling much better.

Dr. Thoung continued seeing me over the next few weeks. I had my arm drained another three times before it was all clear. A total of another 50mls.

It was a long process but finally I felt well and was able to start working on my exercises to get movement and strength back in my arm. It was a relief to get past it but

I couldn't help think that this second time around has not been easy at all.

Treatment

I felt really lucky that this time I didn't need chemo. The lump was 9mm, had been in my body for at least 6 months, but maybe my previous treatment of zoladex and tamoxifen helped enough not to stop cancer but was able to slow the growth.

I went on to have my radiation treatment. Same as the first time, very little had changed in less than 3 years. This time I didn't need to have the tattoos as I already had them. My burns this time were much worse and it started sooner. I was given the same creams to use as before, it took a while but eventually they healed. The side effects of swelling, tiredness, pain I am told will last up to six months. Some days I have energy, other days all I want to do is sleep or rest.

Femara

My oncologist suggested having my ovaries removed. It was an option to think about, she told me there wasn't really any difference between zoladex or ovaries removed, the side effects are the same. She also changed my medication from tamoxifen to Femara. So far, I have only been taking them for a couple of months, the side effects are very similar to tamoxifen, for me. I haven't noticed any significant changes.

Femara (letrozole) is a non-steroidal aromatase inhibitor (lowers estrogen production) used to treat breast cancer in postmenopausal women. It is often given to women who have been taking tamoxifen (Nolvadex, Soltamox) for 5 years. Common side effects of Femara include hot flashes, hair loss, joint/bone/muscle pain, tiredness, unusual sweating or night sweats, nausea, diarrhoea, dizziness, trouble sleeping, drowsiness, weight gain, weakness, flushing (warmth, redness, or tingly feeling), headache, constipation, numbness/tingling/weakness/stiffness in your hand or fingers, or pain in your hand that spreads to your arm, wrist, forearm, or shoulder.

Ovaries

In October I met with a gynaecologist and decided to have my ovaries removed. I would have keyhole surgery. I would be in and out within eight hours, not needing to stay overnight in hospital, that suited me fine.

Of course, the surgery didn't go to plan. I had previously learned that I have developed an allergy to morphine, so am no longer able to have any medication that has morphine in it.
The doctor removed my ovaries, tubes and several cysts. There were complications caused by adhesions from my previous caesarean. The doctor had difficulty

removing my left ovary due to the adhesions, is what I understand. The surgery took a couple of hours longer than expected.

When I woke from the anaesthetic I was in excruciating pain. I have never felt anything like it before. I had pain all down my left side. I was wriggling and crying out. The nurse couldn't give me enough medication to stop the pain. The surgeon was called and it was decided that I would be given a type of anaesthetic because I couldn't have morphine. The doctor explained that it was due to the adhesions that I was feeling so much pain. The doctor said because he knows my pain threshold is high he was hooking me up to a pain machine where I could just press a button whenever I needed relief.

Once my pain was under control and I had the machine attached to me I was moved to a room. I had been in recovery for hours. Jonathan had been waiting all day, expecting me to be out hours earlier. He had no idea and wasn't given any information until I was ready to be moved to a room. I could see how worried he had been, not knowing what was happening or if something was wrong. We both thought I would be home, recovering by now.

I was too drugged and too drowsy to be worried about anything. Staying in hospital overnight didn't worry me at all.

The doctor came in to check on me. He told me not to wait for the pain to be strong before pressing the button. He told me to use it as soon as I felt anything. So that is what I did. I didn't know until later, but Jonathan was also pressing the button for me. I was in and out of sleep all night, every time I woke up I pressed the button and I would go straight back to sleep again. I had a good night. Pain free and worry free thanks to that machine.

The End – For Now ....

I am slowly recovering. It has been a long process.
Initially, I thought it would be easy. I had no idea of the
complications I would face. I have now also developed
esophageal spasms and reflux. When I have an episode I
get such severe pain in my chest that it feels like I am
having a heart attack. I also have scarring on my lungs.
All side effects of radiation.

My left breast is enormous and painful. I have swelling
and fluid pockets in my breast but until the tissue
scarring and swelling subsides, from radiation, I just
have to put up with it.

My right breast continues to get smaller, apparently
there is a name for that too. When I am healthy again I
am able to speak with my surgeon regarding
augmentation. Until then I try to hide away at home.

Both my left and right arms are still weak. I don't have
much movement in my left arm and it is still painful.

I don't know what it's like anymore to live a normal
life. I have forgotten what it feels like to be care free. I
have forgotten what life was like before cancer. I'm not
confident that cancer won't return again. I just live in
hope that the third time will also be my lucky time and
again it will be caught early. I fear that it won't but I try
hard not to think about it. I've learned many things from
having cancer. I have already decided who I will be

telling and who I won't if I am diagnosed again.

 I know how I want to live my life now. None of us are ever certain about how much time we have on Earth but having cancer forces you to realize that it really is a short time. I have wishes that I hope will come true. My biggest wish is of course that this horrible disease never gets me again.

As of Friday 18th March 2016. I am cancer free.

I hope by reading my book it has helped in some way. Whether you can relate to my story or you are newly diagnosed and travelling a similar road.

Please, read my book and pass it on to others, take notice that this horrible disease can get anyone, young or old. Check your breasts regularly. If you notice a change seek advice from your doctor, as soon as possible. If you don't feel comfortable with that doctors opinion then seek a second or third opinion. Never be told you are too young for breast cancer. Never allow a doctor to belittle you. You will be happier when you are treated as you should be.

Don't feel like you have to do this alone. I have found several groups on Facebook for young women with breast cancer and those ladies in these groups are an amazing support. Women from all around the world, all with breast cancer, who understand what you are going through. They are there for you and each other.

There is no ending yet, but let's hope it will be a happy one.

Names of medical staff have been changed for privacy reasons.

www.ingramcontent.com/pod-product-compliance
Lightning Source LLC
Chambersburg PA
CBHW062144280526
45788CB00001B/302